In
Your
Face

Dr Bryan Mendelson is one of the world's leading plastic surgeons. Australian born, he trained at the Mayo Clinic and the New York University Medical Centre and now practices in Melbourne, Australia. He is internationally renowned for his expertise in facial anatomy, and is a former president of the International Society of Aesthetic Plastic Surgery.

Vicki Steggall is a historian who has been writing professionally for twenty-five years, with publications in adult non-fiction and children's literature.

The hidden history of plastic surgery
and why looks matter

In
Your
Face

DR BRYAN MENDELSON

in conjunction with Vicki Steggall

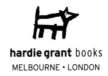

hardie grant books

MELBOURNE · LONDON

Published in 2013 by Hardie Grant Books

Hardie Grant Books (Australia)
Ground Floor, Building 1
658 Church Street
Richmond, Victoria 3121
www.hardiegrant.com.au

Hardie Grant Books (UK)
Dudley House, North Suite
34–35 Southampton Street
London WC2E 7HF
www.hardiegrant.co.uk

Cataloguing-in-Publication data is available from the National Library
of Australia.

In Your Face
ISBN 978 1 74270 123 3

Cover and text design by Christabella Designs
Typeset in Palatino 10.5/17pt by Cannon Typesetting
Cover image courtesy of iStock
Author photograph courtesy of Justin McManus/Fairfax Syndication
Original illustrations by Levent Efe, Melbourne
Colour reproduction by Splitting Image Colour Studio
Printed and bound in Australia by Griffin Press

*In thanks to my wife, Debora, who helped me
to appreciate my abilities and fulfil my potential as
a plastic surgeon, and to my beautiful daughters
Priscilla, Vanessa and Harriet for their love*

Contents

Part 3 Aesthetic plastic surgery today

Introduction

We live our lives behind the most observed and intriguing part of the human body: the face. When I mentioned to people that I was writing a book about the face, they responded with great interest. But when I added that it was also about my specialty—aesthetic plastic surgery—much of their interest turned to disappointment, as if they already knew the end of the story. They'd read about it in magazines or watched it on TV.

It seems that everyone has an opinion on the surgery I perform—surgery for aesthetic (cosmetic) reasons to enhance facial appearance—but very few actually know anything about it. Aesthetic plastic surgery takes place behind closed doors, in a private world designed to protect the patient. This means the human stories remain undisclosed and the media, aware of the general interest in plastic surgery, fills the void with 'information' that bears little relationship to reality. After a lifetime's work in the field, I felt it was time to tell the real story.

Our curiosity about the face and aesthetic surgery is understandable. The human face is as much a psychological space as it is physical, bearing our identity to ourselves and others. It can be an ally throughout life, bringing great ease and opportunity, or it can be an enemy, subverting progress and sapping confidence. It may never have been right to begin with, or, as with ageing, it may no longer feel right. Unlike other animals, we are judged by this mask we live behind and are obliged to accept its relentless deterioration as we age. More frequently than most of us realise, the face can be the cause of silent grief or despair.

It's not surprising, then, that the face has become a metaphor for human life. Every day we get up and face our problems, and if it all goes wrong we face the consequences. We even live in a Facebook world. If we want to hide our identity, we have to hide our face, as everyone from the hangman to the fictional superhero knows well. Without our face, we are also without our self.

That our face is so important—*that it matters*—explains why aesthetic plastic surgery also matters. Of all the surgeries, it's truly about people. Plastic surgery deals with the very soul of the patient, which is why it has been called 'surgery of the psyche'. When a person chooses to have surgery, they're making a decisive statement about their life and how they feel about their identity. Afterwards, they'll change the signals they give out and the responses we give back. Even when the surgery is performed privately and the results are imperceptible to others, they won't be the same person. How can we not be fascinated?

It might seem a very twenty-first-century preoccupation, but the truth is this form of surgery has been with us from ancient times. Ever since we've had the means at our disposal to repair or improve facial appearance we've done so, no matter how basic those means were. Before photography and the media, even before mirrors, people risked their lives with infection and voluntarily submitted to unimaginable pain to have surgery.

Their determination demonstrates that it wasn't about vanity, or the society they lived in, but something more fundamental about being human. The reasons people chose it then are the same reasons people are choosing it today.

When I decided to specialise in aesthetic surgery thirty years ago, I was still too young to really understand how strongly our face influences our lives. At first, I was surprised to see the effect surgery had on people's lives. In the words of a famous surgeon who repaired noses nearly five hundred years ago, I watched it 'buoy up the spirit and help the mind of the afflicted.' Which is a wonderful thing to experience. Three decades on, we've made enormous progress in understanding facial anatomy and facial ageing, which has led to increasingly refined surgical techniques. But, paradoxically, just as our ability to help people has increased so significantly, the reputation of aesthetic surgery within society has plummeted, reduced by media coverage and misinformation to a form of entertainment. This totally misses what my colleagues and I, and our patients, experience every day—and what patients and doctors throughout human civilisation have implicitly understood. In writing this book, I hope to open the doors into the private world of aesthetic plastic surgery, revealing its enduring motivations, some colourful history and characters, and the surgery itself, from the earliest operations to the most advanced procedures we perform today.

One final point. There is a lot of facial surgery performed in society by different doctors, not all of them as trained in surgery as their patients might think. This book is about surgery performed by qualified aesthetic plastic surgeons.

Part 1

The human face

There's nothing as significant as a human face. Nor as eloquent. We can never really know another person, except by our first glance at him. Because, in that glance, we know everything.

Ayn Rand

1

What is the face?

The living face is the most important and
mysterious surface we deal with.
It is the center of our flesh.

Daniel McNeill

Our journey into the human face begins deep under water about 400 million years ago. If it seems a strange and remote place to start our discussion, then we need to be aware that even if we've forgotten our underwater ancestry, our body definitely hasn't. Every aspect of our human face reflects the adaptations that have taken place since our predecessors lived as underwater creatures—gliding around as solitary hunters—and continued as they developed into land-based, upright creatures living in social communities. It's not possible to understand our human face without understanding each of those developmental phases: water life, early life on land, standing upright and communal living. At each stage the face adapted to help its owner survive, and each adaptation has left traces that we can see in the mirror today, as well as deeply hidden structures that a plastic surgeon deals with daily.

Fish face

I've always liked the words of palaeontologist William K Gregory, who stated in 1929 that 'in the face of a shark a man may behold, as in a glass darkly, his own image', reminding us that the twenty-eight bones that form our head and face have each been inherited, in an unbroken line of succession, from an early fish-type creature. If we watch a human embryo develop during its first two months in the womb, we see a kind of time-lapse film of our evolution. At four weeks, the face of a human embryo is fish-like, complete with embryonic gill arches. Two weeks later its face looks no different from a chimpanzee's at the same stage, and it's only at eight weeks that it is sufficiently differentiated to be clearly human.

Think about a shark's face. Its purpose and appearance are essentially as they have been for millions of years. It could be described as a 'mobile food-detecting and food-trapping mask' in front of the brain, a leading edge devoted entirely to survival. It's firm to the touch, allowing it to move fluently through the water. The shark's face is also expressionless, but that isn't a problem as it doesn't need to communicate its emotions to others. Without the need to communicate, the structural demands on its face are very simple: all it has to do is open and close its mouth, and it has one group of jaw-opening muscles located in front of each ear to allow it to do so. Imagine our human face with only enough facial muscles to allow us to gape as we go about our lives.

While our face has evolved so that it looks quite different from the shark's, it still shares the critical, primary function of survival. Consider this description by Gregory of how a shark finds and eats its food. First, its olfactory device (nose) discovers the location of food by its smell (to this day odours reach human noses only in water vapour). Instantly the message is relayed to its brain, causing a reflex rotation of its eyes, allowing it to locate the prey. Then, the final act: a convulsive expansion of the jaw before it snaps shut to trap the prey. Are we really so different, eating breakfast? With today's focus on the appearance of the human face, it's easy to forget that its primary function is not to look nice but to enable us to survive by taking in air, and finding and eating food. When we think about it in this way, we can see through today's superficial arrangements of hairstyles and makeup, and look more deeply, to the basic survival functions beneath.

One final observation about the shark. Its face ages extraordinarily well—quite unlike the human face. For that it can thank its simple anatomical structure and that single set of jaw-opening muscles. We humans pay a price for our highly mobile faces—something we'll return to many times in this book.

From fish to human

Unlike the shark, we didn't remain in the sea, and the firm, expressionless face of a fish was no longer suitable for our needs. We developed our own variant on the general positioning of eyes, nose and mouth. All animals have their own version of this configuration, because it's functional and it works. But, as Charles Darwin (1809–1882) observed, survival is linked not just to functionality but also to the capacity to change; we can see how facial change has occurred in the multiplicity of animal faces on earth, each using the same basic configuration but evolved to meet specific needs.

The faces of our earliest land-based ancestors were covered with protective plate-type armour, like a reptile's, and these ancestors lived close to the ground. In time, the facial surface became more supple and leathery, but vision was yet to develop and tactile whiskers compensated; the remnants of these are evident in humans today as eyebrows. Later, muscle started to cover the amour, beginning with the neck and creeping upwards until it spread across the entire face, while the bony mask sank deeper below the surface. This early muscular covering, which originated in the neck, is called the primitive platysma and is still with us as the broad, flat muscle layer that covers our neck and lower face. With time, the parts of the primitive platysma on the face that were not being used atrophied, leaving small islands of effective muscle situated in key parts of the face wherever movement was required. In particular, the function of the facial muscles was to control the coverings of the eyes and mouth (the lids and lips over the two main apertures of the facial skeleton), as well as the sides of the nose and, at that stage, the ears (which is why some people can still waggle their ears). As these islands of muscle developed, the possibility of facial expression arose.

Our next stage of evolution—as we ascended to the highest order of mammals, the primates—meant moving above the ground, into the safety of trees. As a result, reliance on the sense of smell diminished and sight became more important.

Sharp vision and coordination were required for these greater computational demands, so the brain enlarged to provide for this, while the once-mobile nose and prominent ears became smaller. Our eyes moved forwards, allowing them to function as a pair and to provide the stereoscopic sight needed for swinging on one branch and grasping the branch ahead—impossible without accurate eye-to-hand coordination. The price of failure on a high trapeze can be costly.

Standing upright changed the position of our ancestors' faces. They needed a distinct neck, to allow the top joint between the vertebrae and the skull to rotate downwards by as much as ninety degrees to compensate for the vertical position of the body. We now have a useful neck, but how much human suffering has resulted from this relatively recent adaptation! The eye developed a 'sweet spot' on the retina to give refined, sharp vision perfectly suited to the way in which humans communicate, by looking directly into the central 'zone of expression' on each other's faces: the area around the eyes and lips.

As early humans developed beyond the great-ape stage, their need to communicate with each other also developed. As a small, not especially fast animal, they benefited from harnessing the power of working communally in a number of ways, such as hunting. This required the complex facial mobility and communication that set humans apart from other animals. Facial expression became critical to survival in the group, but, on the other hand, the face was no longer so necessary for fighting—hands and weapons took over that role. For the human face it was a constant process of change and adaptation, with communication becoming an increasingly important function.

Our cousins, the great apes, can communicate using their faces but the difference is that they are physically limited to large, mass movements. We modern humans have developed facial expression to such a degree that we have a large range of finely nuanced expressions. Even a slightly raised eyebrow or a narrowing of the lips has meaning, and only humans could have been entertained by silent movies, where one person's facial movements are interpreted and understood by thousands of others. This, of course, has required our face to develop a complex anatomy to deliver precise movement so we can signal what we are thinking and express the wide range of emotions and psychological states we feel. But this mobility also has to be balanced with structural stability, for we still need to retain control over the extent of the movement. It's that degree of mobility and control that our simian cousins don't possess. A monkey's face is fixed to the skeleton by tough, sinewy ligaments that prohibit small movements of the facial muscles and therefore make lively expressions—necessary for true communication—impossible. This is something I found for myself when dissecting a monkey's face, which turned out to be very hard work!

It is only in the last 100,000 years that the modern human face has developed and humans have stopped looking so ape-like—as human survival extended beyond the primary requirements of breathing and feeding to include such finely balanced communication that at times a human's safety could depend on how another human reads their expression. We are, after all, one of the very few animals that chooses to live in large groups of mostly complete strangers. As we ascended the evolutionary ladder, the ape's huge mouth, strong teeth, receding chin and broad, flat nose gave way to a narrow, projecting nose and small mouth, a flatter face, weak jaws with reduced projection of the teeth, a high, rounded forehead or brow, and a projecting chin, a feature unique to the human. The functions of the eyelids and mouth developed to take us to the next level of expression. Our eyes and mouth are each surrounded by a sphincter muscle, which gives us precise and important control over their movements, and because the surface of our eyes is unprotected, the aperture formed around them by the lids is kept small and also moves with the eyes. It's a fantastic system, so finely calibrated that when it goes seriously wrong, for instance with burn victims, it can lead not just to loss of expression but to loss of the ability of the lid to protect the eyeball itself—the two related survival functions of the eyelid.

Another important change, deeper in our anatomy, concerned the attachment of the facial muscles. In most other animals the facial muscles are attached only to the soft tissues of the face, but in humans this has developed further, to the point where most of the muscles are also attached to the underlying bone. It's almost as if they reached out to grasp the bone in preference to the tissue. Why is this important? Attachment to the bone gives more precision to movements of the muscle, and precise muscle control is the mechanism that enables precise facial expression. This attachment is not exclusive to humans but develops progressively in the higher species, according to functional need, reaching its greatest degree in the human face.

It shows how fundamentally the face has evolved to meet the demands inherent in creating visible expression, that is, expression that can show up clearly on its surface: the skin.

Some tribal groups around the world do have slightly different attachments in their facial muscles. For example, in Australian Indigenous peoples the malaris muscle, which lifts the top of the cheek, extends further down the face than it does in other humans. In the classical era of anatomy, from the 1880s to the 1930s, it was fashionable to study anatomical differences between racial groups, especially in those who varied from a more 'general' (that is, European) appearance, to discover what advantages or limitations their anatomies might inherently possess. Such small variations demonstrate how various groups of Homo sapiens have evolved slightly differently around the shared imperative of communication.

The fantastical face

The human face, with its myriad expressions and variations, has fascinated artists and writers for centuries. We have only to think of Leonardo da Vinci's *Mona Lisa* (c. 1503–06) or Edvard Munch's *The Scream* (1893) for examples of facial expressions depicted in such a way as to cause unending analysis and speculation. Edmond Rostand's *Cyrano de Bergerac* (1897), better known to contemporary audiences for its adaptation as the film *Roxanne* (1987), tackled facial difference: the protagonist's huge nose and facial ugliness led him to believe that he was unable to dream of love even with an ugly woman. His face was more important in the course of his life than his heart or intellect.

Another wonderful example of the face in literature is found in Thomas de Quincey's *Confessions of an English Opium Eater* (1821), in which we are made aware of the face's ability to form the ultimate nightmare, haunting and tormenting. De Quincey describes the 'fierce chemistry' of his dreams, which are fuelled by opium yet start off mildly, with architectural themes—cities and palaces, pavilions and towers in the sky—then change to watery subjects—lakes and silvery expanses, seas and oceans. However, there follows a 'tremendous change', which stays with him and gives abiding torment: the appearance of the human face.

> But now that which I have called the tyranny of the
> human face began to unfold itself ... now it was that upon

the rocking waters of the ocean the human face began to appear; the sea paved with innumerable faces upturned to the heavens—faces imploring, wrathful, despairing, surged upwards by thousands, by myriads, by generations, by centuries: my agitation was infinite; my mind tossed and surged with the ocean.

Aptly, the catalyst for De Quincey's addiction to opium was the need to alleviate pain resulting from severe bouts of trigeminal neuralgia—acute facial pain—a condition well known to drive sufferers to despair and addiction.

End result

So, what is the human face? It's a survival surface, in the primary senses of breathing and feeding, and also in the secondary sense of enabling us to live in our more recent, communal world. It's also, as we will see in the following chapters, a player in that world, its outward appearance affecting not only those who see it but the human who lives behind it. For humans, the importance of the face has gone far beyond that of other animals, being the signifier of each person's individuality amid the group—to themselves and others. Our face contributes to the person we are, and if we were given another we would be someone else, both to ourselves and to others. Our lives would, most probably, be quite different—even with so seemingly insignificant a variation of just a few millimetres of nose length. It makes you wonder how human evolution will handle the increasingly important social and psychological dimensions of facial appearance and, as a result of this, what the human face will look like in another 10,000 years.

2

Expression

An eye can threaten like a loaded and levelled
gun, or it can insult like hissing or kicking; or, in its
altered mood, by beams of kindness, it can make
the heart dance for joy.

Ralph Waldo Emerson

People are fascinated by the power of facial expression; there are even television shows devoted to the subject. Is this person lying or telling the truth? Are they truly expressing an emotion or are they simply acting? It makes good television, but out in the real world it's not a game; it's something we rely upon to gauge almost every social situation we find ourselves in. Sometimes it's even life and death.

Author Malcolm Gladwell tells the story of a Los Angeles policeman who pulled over a sports car late one night to be confronted by a young man leaping out of the passenger-side door and aiming a gun at him. For a moment, both stood with guns pointing at each other, but the policeman, instead of shooting, chose to hold fire. Against all logic he went with his gut reaction, which was induced by the expression on the young man's face. He was right, and the other man backed down. The policeman's life depended on the truth that was conveyed in a fraction of a second by a facial expression. Fortunately, his ability to read faces and his years of experience with people in difficult situations led him to the right conclusion. Most of us are not as good at reading other people's faces as he was.

The face as entertainment

Facial expression is often used to provide entertainment, particularly in the theatre and by comedians. Some actors develop an astonishing capacity for expression. In the eighteenth century, British actor David Garrick became famous for being able to rotate at speed through the facial expressions for nine emotions—joy, tranquillity, surprise, astonishment, sadness, despondency, fear, horror and despair. And in the eighteenth and nineteenth centuries, when other forms of entertainment were thin on the ground, grinning or grotesque face-making contests were regularly held in parts of the United Kingdom. Angus Trumble, in *A Brief History of the Smile*, describes these events, which certainly demonstrate that smiling and grinning are two very different uses of the human face. One 'angry grin' competitor was said by *The Spectator* in September 1711 to have produced a grin so successful in its object that he 'made half a dozen women miscarry'. Another competitor was described as having such a complicated grin that it left the spectators astonished. They would have awarded him the win

> had it not been proved by one of his antagonists, that he
> had practised with verjuice for some days before, and had
> a crab found upon him at the very time of grinning.

He was consequently disqualified for cheating. The ultimate winner, a cobbler, produced several original face distortions, including giving the appearance of a spout, a baboon and a pair of nutcrackers. It was surely an accomplished performance, since not only did he win a gold ring, but a 'country wench' was so impressed by his feats that she married him the next week, having spurned his advances for the preceding five years.

For reasons that are not entirely clear, extreme grinning could be fatal. In June 1804, *The Times* in London reported that

> a grinning-match lately took place at Bridlington, for a quantity of tobacco. There were three competitors for the prize, all of whom were speedily seized with the most painful symptoms, in consequence of their violent contortions, and two of them died in a few days; the third lies dangerously ill.

Face-distorting competitions, known as gurning competitions, are still held in certain countries, so their fascination remains. An ugly face competition, or *Concurso de Feos*, is part of the Great Week celebrations in Bilbao, with photographs of some of the more grotesque expressions appearing in the international press. The World Gurning Championship is held annually in Cumbria, in which contestants attempt to produce the most distorted facial expression, some even having their teeth removed to enhance their 'gurn'.

Facial expression is a critical attribute of being human, and the basic language of facial expression is universal, shared by humans across the planet even though we have different cultures, gestures and spoken languages. It's the cornerstone of human communication, an innate part of us. Charles Darwin was one of the first to study these similarities of expression, which he observed during his extensive travels as a young man. In 1866, he decided to test whether expression truly is universal among humans. He sent out a questionnaire to people who dealt with remote tribal communities or with communities that had experienced little contact with European culture. The questionnaire contained sixteen questions specifically designed to find out whether the same facial expressions were shared by all humans. If they were, this would show that expressions are innate and instinctive to humans, thereby providing further evidence that all humans share a common ancestor.

Darwin's questions were specific and included 'Is astonishment expressed by the eyes and mouth being opened wide, and by the eyebrows being raised?' and 'Is contempt expressed by a slight protrusion of the lips and by a turning up of the nose, with a slight expiration?' He received thirty-six replies, from China, Borneo, India, Sri Lanka, Egypt and the United States. Australia provided thirteen responses from people who lived among the country's Aboriginal peoples. The respondents were generous in their details, and these, plus Darwin's own observations and those of the French neurologist Guillaume-Benjamin-Amand Duchenne de Boulogne, suggested that expression is indeed universal. This formed the basis of Darwin's book *The Expression of the Emotions in Man and Animals* (1872).

A century later, psychologist Paul Ekman, a key name in the field, was so convinced that Darwin was wrong—that expressions were not universal but cultural—that he didn't even bother to read Darwin's book. But after spending six months examining thirty metres of film of people from the isolated cultures of the Highlands of Papua New Guinea he made the surprised observation that he 'never saw an unfamiliar expression'. He proposed that six key expressions are universal:

enjoyment, sadness, anger, fear, disgust and surprise. Ekman then visited the Highlands in person to test this theory. He took with him pictures of different human faces to show the villagers he met. He would tell them a story, such as about someone losing a child, and ask them to point to the picture of the most relevant expression. The results were clear-cut for happiness, anger, disgust and sadness. Fear and surprise were not clearly distinguished from each other, but they were distinguished from the first four.

The importance of a true smile

In his work *The Varieties of Human Facial Expression* (1997), Dutch artist Arthur Elsenaar managed to create 4096 expressions in thirty-two minutes by electrically stimulating his facial muscles. Out of all these expressions, only one was seen to denote 'nothing', or to be a meaning-less expression. This suggests, as writer Daniel McNeill has said, that 'our face is constantly communicating because, unlike other forms of communication such as speech, it is never turned off'. It's something politicians learn: if they wear a smirk or a shifty expression, even when not speaking, they will be judged for it, but if they smile people will like them.

The human smile triggered the historical investigation of facial expressions. Guillaume-Benjamin-Amand Duchenne de Boulogne (1806–1875) was a French neurologist. Using an old man described as an 'old almshouse denizen' who was (allegedly and hopefully) impervious to pain as his 'guinea pig', Duchenne applied electrical currents to the facial muscles in order to map out their movements and the expressions they create. When he looked at smiles, he found that simply pulling up the corners of the mouth (using the zygomatic major muscle) did not create an expression of enjoyment, but when the muscles around the eyes (the orbicularis oculi muscles) were also contracted, joy was expressed. Without true joy, the orbicularis oculi did not contract, leaving a mouth-only smile. Duchenne described it beautifully: the muscles around the eyes are put into play only 'by the sweet emotions of the soul', while their 'inertia, in smiling, unmasks a false friend'.

Daniel McNeill has suggested that the film made of this experiment is one of our earliest maps of human expression. We now know there are dozens of different smiles, but only a smile created by true pleasure is able to create contractions in the ring of muscle around the eyes. It's interesting that these tiny contractions, only just perceptible to an observer, are for most of us entirely involuntary; only about 10 per cent of people can consciously create them. Unless you are experiencing the joyous pre-conditions for a true smile, you are unlikely to create one. Even a ten-month-old baby will give a true smile to its mother but a lesser smile to strangers.

This explains why sometimes when a person smiles at us we don't get the corresponding feeling that they're actually pleased to see us, while other smiles light up the room. It also means that at social events when we make our face ache from smiling, the likelihood is that nobody is actually convinced by our efforts. Happily married couples greet each other at the end of the day with 'Duchenne' smiles, but in unhappy marriages such smiles are absent. Furthermore, according to Paul Eckman, people who give Duchenne smiles experience more happiness and lower blood pressure, and are reported by friends and spouses to be happy in general: an everyday example of the importance of expression for our emotional wellbeing.

Ekman found that the human face can produce more than ten thousand different expressions, using varying combinations of muscle movements. Of these, around three thousand have meaning; that is, they are linked to emotions. In 1978, he produced an 'atlas' of the face known as the Facial Action Coding System, which shows through words, film and photographs how to measure facial movements in anatomical terms. This has been used by animators, police and a host of other people interested in analysing facial expression.

We also use our facial muscles to animate or replace conversation. This includes actions like a wink for shared experience, a raised eyebrow for cynicism and a smile or a nod for agreement, all of which can convey information along with or in place of the spoken word. Ekman called this paralanguage. Unlike expression, paralanguage is more likely to be culturally determined; for example, you would need to be careful with raising an eyebrow or winking in some cultures. Paralanguage can also be quite extensive: Ekman isolated sixty facial communications common in the United States.

Grins

The grin, especially one that's misplaced, demonstrates the power of facial expression to affect us on a deep psychological level. In 1869, the French writer Victor Hugo created in *The Man Who Laughs* the story of a boy, Gwynplaine, whose face was mutilated to produce the appearance of a perpetual grin, a horrifying version of a clown's mask. This was carried out by a group of wanderers who disfigured children and used them as entertainment from which they derived an income. The repugnant idea is made worse by the fact that a grin suggests youthful merriment, when the boy's circumstances clearly caused the very opposite emotion. His expression has an easily understood meaning, so when it appears in the wrong place this adds to the horror of the mutilation and instills in the reader a deep sense of unease. Since Hugo's time, a vast array of adaptations, including movies and plays, have sprung from this idea of the misplaced grin—such is the ghoulish fascination that it provokes.

We might today compare this with Heath Ledger's depiction of The Joker in Christopher Nolan's *The Dark Knight*, his face grinning impassively even as he inflicts terror and death on those around him. It's the face of a madman: we can't read his emotions and suspect he has none. There's no traction for us to make contact with him and communicate, which is so critical for humans. His lack of expression and huge grinning lips distort everything we unconsciously rely upon facial expression to tell us, lending a Gothic horror to every scene he appears in and creating an unforgettable facial image.

Expression and emotion

There is an astonishing link between facial expression and emotion. Most of us instinctively know that expression reflects emotion. Darwin, while travelling on a train, watched an elderly woman with a 'comfortable but absorbed expression' in the seat opposite suddenly rotate through a series of subtle facial expressions. He saw a slight drawing down at the corners of her mouth, which he initially thought might be meaningless, but this was followed by her eyes filling with tears, leading him to suspect that she had recollected a painful occurrence. With suppression of her muscles she withheld her responses, presumably because she was in public. Not a word was spoken, but Darwin saw these fleeting expressions and was able to interpret them. Today, we could plot the sequence of emotions using magnetic resonance imaging (MRI) technology. It would start with an electrical impulse fired in the woman's brain as a result of recalling grief, and this would instantly translate into corresponding muscle contractions across the face. But Darwin, well before the era of MRI, observed the woman with amazement. 'The links are indeed wonderful which connect cause and effect in giving rise to various expressions on the human countenance.'

Interestingly, the link between emotion and expression is two-way: when we consciously produce a particular facial expression, it feeds back into the brain and can actually trigger the emotion we were expressing. If you hold a pencil horizontally between your teeth, creating a slight smile expression, your emotional response to the world will lift; in research, people have found cartoons funnier when they do this. Conversely, if you put the pencil between your pursed lips, so it sticks out in front of you creating a slight frown, you are likely to experience a greater response to upsetting pictures. It confirms the old adage, from an era well before psychological research, that if you smile you'll feel better. These simple but striking examples show that our face can be used as a sort of switch to change emotions. Darwin wrote that 'the free expression by outward signs of an emotion intensifies it … He who does not control the signs of fear will experience fear in a greater degree'. Many of us have experienced this: we know that keeping a calm face helps to retain the feeling of calmness in situations of fear or frustration.

Expressing emotion empowers communication and can even elicit a response that is beneficial for us. For example, an expression of grief can evoke sympathy from others; in fact, Paul Eckman's research proved that we are so attuned to grief that we even feel sadness just looking at a picture of someone with a melancholy expression. And Darwin observed that sympathy with another person's distress produces tears more easily than our own personal distress. In fact, one of the ways we engage with others is to unconsciously mimic their facial expressions as they talk, for instance smiling when they do, expressing grief or joy along with them. It goes well beyond just the contagion of laughter, which we all know well. Mimicking facial expression builds the intensity and involvement between the speaker and listener. If we withhold our expression, we remain more detached and have less investment in the other person's viewpoint or the experience they relate. Research into facial mimicry—and body mimicry—has grown enormously in the past ten years, demonstrating a wide range of situations in which humans unconsciously use mimicry to build rapport and influence the decisions of others. Amongst the many studies, one asked students to listen to another's story and determine whether the person was telling the truth. If the students listened impassively, without mimicking the other person's facial expressions, they were significantly more successful at determining if that person was lying or not. By withholding their facial expression, they kept emotional distance and didn't buy into the other person's emotions.

Research presented at 'Neuroscience 2012' showed that automatic facial mimicking is a social behaviour that plays a role in our ability to learn and understand, as well as create rapport. It revealed new connections between mimicry and its underlying brain circuitry, showing that the automatic movement of our facial muscles, to reflect the movement of the facial muscles of the person speaking to us, has greater meaning than we might have supposed. We discern meaning through facial mimicry via the use of 'ever more specialised' brain circuits that provide us with feedback, according to Martha Farah of the University of Pennsylvania. Mimicry even has status connotations, as a powerful person can suppress a smile towards other high-status people, while lower-status people tend to mimic everyone's smile. We also subconsciously mimic when we try to interpret others' ambiguous smiles, using it as another 'tool' to try to understand what the other person is really thinking when it's not clear by their smile alone.

A life with no smile

Why are specific basic facial expressions understood by all of us to be a signal of our emotional state? The brow alone is the site of many of these responses. Why, when we're struggling with any form of difficulty, mental or physical, do we contract our brow? Or raise our eyebrows when we experience fear? Unfortunately, we don't yet know the entire answer to these questions. However, what we do know is that the brow is highly wired for emotion, so using our brow is both an automatic response of the nervous system stemming from deep in our past, as well as a communication to others. It's our muscle's response to strong emotions: something we once had to learn but that is now as involuntary as our heart's fast-beating response to danger.

In fact, as we've already observed, we're better at the involuntary production of facial expressions than we are at reading them. The policeman who decided not to shoot was more proficient at reading someone's emotions from their face than most of us, which was fortunate for him—few except the most basic facial expressions are reliably understood between people. We've all experienced instances when we've misread someone's face and therefore what was being communicated.

Frowning is one expression that most humans understand as negative in some way, and, like most human facial communication, it starts with the first weeks of the mother–baby relationship. Darwin described the frown as the earliest and almost sole expression of babies, who, when they are as young as one week old, precede their screaming fits with a slight brow contraction. And when a baby suffers discomfort, little frowns 'may be seen incessantly passing like shadows' over their face, even though these may not be followed by crying.

The opposite of this—the smile—also develops early in a baby's life, usually by the time they are eight weeks old, and this is another expression understood by most humans, this time as showing pleasure.

Even though we may occasionally misread others' facial communication, the use of facial expression to communicate and amplify our emotions has become integral to our existence as humans. To spend an hour in the company of others and remain completely without expression would be very difficult, both for us and for those around us. But there are some people who do live like that, who are unable to use their faces to communicate, and their experience provides the ultimate test of just how important facial expression is. These are the people who suffer from Moebius syndrome, which produces total or near-total facial paralysis from birth. This can include a permanently open mouth as well as unblinking eyes and limited eye movement (only up and down), which effectively prohibits any sideways glances or eye-related communication. On the Moebius Syndrome Foundation's website, the mother of a sufferer explained the implications of the syndrome for her child's social and psychological future: 'Your baby will never smile, never have facial expression, never blink his eyes, never move his eyes laterally. Your baby is sentenced to a life with no SMILE'. Kathleen Bogart, a psychology researcher who has the syndrome, described to *The New York Times* in April 2010 her experience of struggling to communicate to others without the ability to produce movements with her face: 'Stripped of the facial expression, the emotion just dies there, unshared. It just dies'.

As a human, the need to share emotion is so strong that we now even use facial expression as a way of sharing our emotions when using the written word to communicate. The ubiquitous emoticon—the simple parenthesis and colon—when added to an email allows the sender to convey their feelings along with the message, ensuring that the recipient more truly understands the intent behind the words. Emoticons might sometimes be annoying, but their popularity is testament to our urge to share emotion and not just convey information. And what better way to do this than to send a facial expression? To imperil a person's facial expression is to imperil their ability to move through human society as a normal person, and to interact comfortably. For Moebius sufferers, this is their daily reality, but it's also a criticism levelled at poor-quality facial surgery or the overuse of botox. With everything we now know about the importance of facial expression, and the ongoing research that is uncovering more information almost weekly, it's a serious charge.

Sharing a smile

I'm often surprised at the stereotypes attached to the desire to improve the appearance of the human face. They give short shrift to what is really going on. To me the motives are more complex, both more appealing and more endearing.

In 2007 I had an accident that damaged my mouth and my ability to smile. In square-inch terms the damage wasn't major, but it meant that I lost my open smile—and in doing so I lost a critical part of myself. Until that happened, I hadn't known that in some important way my smile defined me.

I like being open with people, to focus on our interaction and feel the rapport growing. But my damaged face changed my focus. I found I was unable to look at others in the same open, unselfconscious way. I no longer felt like a clear vessel. There was a barrier and that was my sadness at not being able to smile warmly and openly. I no longer felt myself so capable of enjoying people, and I no longer felt okay.

Sometimes we forget that human beings are extraordinary, sensing creatures. Part of being human is to respond to that which is harmonious: our eyes linger longer where there is visual harmony and grace. We respond to the whole. Eye contact between people gives us emotional sustenance and I believe we are actually nourished by soft eye contact that lingers gently.

I'm sure there are some souls who see their appearance as a currency they can use to gain power in human relationships. But the issue isn't appearance at all. It goes well beyond that. I believe it's about rapport, freedom. Relationships. And, most importantly, it's about being looked on with gentleness.

3

Looking at faces

There's no art to find the mind's
construction in the face.

William Shakespeare

As we have seen, thanks to evolution the need to communicate has changed our face, literally. Its primary purpose is still survival—seeing, eating and breathing—but its secondary function as a hard-working communicator is also critical, and that role starts from the moment we're born, with facial recognition. One of the first things a newborn baby can do is recognise its mother; from between just twelve and thirty-six hours after birth an infant makes more sucking noises when seeing a video of its mother than when shown a video of a stranger. This early facial recognition a full year before most are able to walk shows why so much human activity is based around appearance. Soon babies delight their parents with a range of expressions: they can show happiness between six weeks and three months, anger between three and seven months and fear between five and nine months. They use their face to communicate even when they don't know they have one—which is truly fascinating.

We're hardwired for facial recognition: it's a significant part of our brain's work. When we see a new face, our brain translates what we're seeing into a neural code—an advanced form of pattern recognition. So much of our brain is dedicated to this exercise that it has been described by researchers at the University of Texas as 'the most finely tuned system we have'. This largely unconscious process occurs without our active effort except in situations such as parties, when we need to try to remember everyone's name. Our eyes feed the information to our brain by scanning rapidly across the face we're looking at, choosing key points, usually starting with the mouth, then moving up to the eyes. Along the way, our eyes will stop at anything unexpected, like a scar or a mole, almost as if they have a mind of their own. We've all experienced consciously trying *not* to look at something distracting on another person's face only to feel our eyes inexorably drawn back towards it. If something doesn't look right, we notice it. We may not be able to explain what's wrong, but human eyes are highly sensitive to a mismatch between what they expect to find in a face and what they see, especially in the critical area around the eyes and mouth, where we focus our attention.

For the person we are meeting, even the smallest deviation in our eye contact in that first moment destroys the character of the interaction. It's this loss of steady eye contact that people with a facial abnormality feel most keenly, even when their abnormality is very small. Research shows that 'facially aware people' desire the same unflinching eye contact that most people enjoy almost unthinkingly, and the loss of it makes their social encounters uncomfortable. Our predisposition to notice deviations from the norm effectively reminds them of their problem. Frances Cooke MacGregor, a social scientist who studied the psychological effects of facial abnormalities, found that the response of others—that momentary subconscious movement of their eyes—creates a burden even when not meant unkindly. In fact, her study found that this reactive behaviour of others created more suffering and damage to the self-esteem of people with facial abnormalities than that caused by seeing their reflection in the mirror. They experience this unavoidably going about their day-to-day lives, travelling, shopping, working or just walking along a street.

For those who brave social encounters while feeling facially aware, the effort can be exhausting. A woman with a facial paralysis affecting her eyelids explained it clearly: 'My facial appearance detracts from what I say'. Another observed, 'I must pretend to be gay at any price ... I must win people with my charm or create an atmosphere which will distract others from my disfigurement'.

Ultimately the emotional fatigue resulting from the cumulative effect of other people's scrutiny leads to a loss of confidence and a loss of desire for any sort of social encounter.

Physiognomy

When we first meet people we make assumptions about them based on their facial appearance. Our assessment may not endure, but judging people by their faces is part of being human. We all do it, even if, just as we attempt not to stare at blemishes, we try not to. Storytellers have long known the importance of the face, using facial description to convey personality. In most cultures there is a 'code' of stylised descriptions and illustrations that convey to the listener or reader the character of the person portrayed: the crumpled face and crooked nose of the witch; the shifty eyes of the sly, deceitful person; the large, round eyes and rosebud mouth of the innocent heroine. No-one brought up in the Western tradition could see an illustration of a witch's face and mistake it for a heroine, or see a beautiful young woman and think she was a thief. Today's artists continue to convey character through facial features: if they want to draw someone vicious, they don't give them a button nose.

At various times throughout history, judgement by face has been considered a serious scientific exercise, known as 'physiognomy'. The ability of a study of the face to determine character was widely accepted by the ancient Greeks—Pythagoras and Aristotle were two exponents—and it was an early university subject in England before being outlawed by Henry VIII, along with palmistry.

Probably the best known physiognomist was Swiss pastor and author Johann Kaspar Lavater (1741–1801), who wrote at length on the subject. For him, it was a matter of science that each person's facial features mirrored the inner person; he believed that a face at rest showed 'character betrayed', so if the parts of the face were understood they would indicate 'the signs of the powers and inclinations of men'. He defined physiognomy as 'the science or knowledge of the correspondence between the external and internal man, the visible superficies and the invisible contents'. He considered it self-evident that as no two faces are the same and no two people are the same there must be a functioning link between them. His theories were immensely popular.

Lavater believed that as we all practise physiognomy, even if unconsciously, every time we meet a stranger there must be an innate understanding that it is possible to gauge a person's character from doing so. Is there anyone, he asked, 'who does not, more or less, the first time he encounters a stranger, observe, estimate, compare and judge him, according to appearances?' He went so far as to ask 'what knowledge is there, of which man is capable, that is not founded on the exterior?' In other words, how can we make sense of the world without observation forming the first step to understanding? It's a reasonable question, but Lavater took it further, which is where today we probably part company with his theories. He believed that it was possible to divine from the face the morality of the person within. Each part of the face played a role: the forehead mirrored the person's understanding, the nose and cheeks their morality and sensibility, their mouth and chin their 'animal' life. The eyes were the summary and centre of the whole. By reading these sections of the face one could form a picture of the person's moral life.

It was not a simple process: Lavater listed one hundred rules of physiognomy, covering everything from ambiguous thinkers to warts. Even animals were included in Lavater's physiognomy: their external features reflected the animal within, such as cruelty in the snout and eyes of the tiger, feebleness of outline in the sloth, and nobility and pride expressed by a horse. The crocodile, he said, 'like other creatures, but more visibly and infallibly than others, in all its parts, outlines and points, has physiognomy that cannot be mistaken'. From its face he deduced that a crocodile is debased, despicable, knotty, obstinate, wicked, void of all love and affection and a 'fiend incarnate'.

Electing chins

The chin is especially important for politicians. Research in 2010 showed that we are biologically predisposed to accept or reject political candidates according to their facial attributes, and the largest advantage comes from having a strong chin, which we take as denoting competence. Trustworthiness is also an important attribute and is assumed to be part of a person's character if they bear a slight smile. A combination of a strong chin and a slight smile gives the voter a feeling of confidence in a candidate. Originally based on the reaction of Princeton students to campaign portraits of politicians, the correlation between a strong chin, a confident smile and politicians winning elections has been confirmed in several countries, adding currency to Johann Kaspar Lavater's words that we are all influenced by physiognomy—even today.

Focusing back on the human world, Lavater bravely tried to answer an interesting question: why is there so much ugliness in people, and so little true beauty? It's something we've probably all wondered at times. His answer was that there is a tendency for virtue to beautify and for vice to deform. In an era before genetic inheritance was understood, Lavater explained that one person's degeneracy, for instance, affected both the individual and their ensuing generations, leading to 'bloated, depressed, turgid, stupid, disfigured, and haggard features'. Many people ridiculed Lavater's ideas, but he had a useful explanation for this: he claimed that secretly they did believe him but were fearful that if physiognomy gained legitimacy their true selves would be revealed to others.

British artist William Hogarth (1697–1764) pondered the same question of the relationship between looks and morality, but from an artist's perspective. He posed the question, 'How did the ancient sculptors, faced with the task of producing a likeness of a deity, portray their subject's greater than human wisdom?' It's an interesting question. The ancient sculptors did what seems naturally correct and chose beauty as a means to convey this great wisdom. We now accept that beauty is a widely understood physical metaphor for morality and wisdom, although for an artist or sculptor it does have its limitations: as Hogarth observed, there are many more ways to depict moral deficiency through facial features than there are to convey moral superiority.

Hogarth felt that humans naturally associate a person's facial features with their inner being.

> We can scarce help forming some particular conception of the person's mind we are observing, even before we receive information by any other means … We all concur at first sight, when we see a downright idiot, an honest or good natured man, or a cunning rogue. Similarly we seldom fail, when looking at kings, murderers, saints and heroes to link their looks with their deeds.

However, he also realised that facial features can be deceiving and that we can be fooled by a face. He gave the example of men hiding foolish or wicked minds behind handsome faces: they betray themselves only by word or deed. A bad man, he said, can, if he manages the movements of his facial muscles sufficiently, teach those muscles to 'contradict his heart'. Hogarth stressed the truth of the adage *fronti nulla fides* ('you can't put any faith in appearances'), believing that physiognomists placed 'too great a stress on outward show'.

Governments and faces

Governments are well aware of the importance of facial appearance. Any government wanting to demonstrate its success will show the faces of its people, smiling and happy, in its promotional material, as a subliminal demonstration that it has their safety and wellbeing in hand and that they can show their faces freely as individuals. In contrast, totalitarian regimes are depicted by writers and painters as those whose people do not have individual faces, or at least do not dare show them. In his famous futuristic novel *Nineteen Eighty-Four* (1949), George Orwell described a future in which human identity is smashed beneath the state, leaving a world of terror and treachery. To describe this world, one of the characters uses the telling words 'if you want a picture of the future, imagine a boot stamping on a human face—forever'.

Do faces matter?

This question irritates many people who feel, quite understandably, that our face and looks don't matter at all. They agree with Hogarth that judging someone on looks alone is as unworthy an exercise as judging a book by its cover—something we are warned against as children. In many ways they have a point: clearly, a person matters more than their face does. And the idea that there is any actual science in the relationship between facial appearance and a person's character or moral worth has certainly fallen out of favour. But the reality is—and research tells us—that our face *does* matter. A high forehead persists in being linked to intellect, and an under-pronounced chin with weakness of character. Intellect is also often correlated (perhaps unconsciously) with beauty. Studies show male educators give essays higher marks if they think the female writer is attractive, teachers assume that good-looking students are more intelligent, and students from primary school to university rate attractive teachers as being more organised, friendlier and better overall. There is no logical basis to suspect that chin size indicates anything other than the size of our parents' chins, but we are clearly wired to think differently about this. Frequently, such assessments affect the ways in which we interact with the people we meet or the opinion we have of them. We see personality in facial features and act accordingly, until our initial judgement is proved or disproved. There are evolutionary advantages in being able to make an instant assessment of a stranger based on perceptions about facial structure, just as there are with expression. It might just keep us safe. But for someone born with a face that doesn't reflect their personality, this can mean being constantly misjudged. As we will see later, a significant mismatch between how a person looks and their real personality can also bring patients to the plastic surgeon.

Physiognomy is still with us, whether we're just meeting someone for the first time at a party, instantly assessing strangers' faces to see if they pose a threat to our safety, or deciding if a politician is competent enough to earn our vote. And because the face presents itself first, before we have a chance to reveal anything else about ourselves, there are probably many situations in which faces matter even more than what lies beneath. In today's fast-moving world, geared to fleeting appearances and instant reactions, it is almost certainly so.

4

The right face

In every man's heart there is a secret nerve
that answers to the vibrations of beauty.

Christopher Morley

As we saw in the preceding chapter, it can be argued that physiognomy is still with us today, although not formally practised, as we make unconscious assessments about people such as politicians based on their appearance. Nowhere is this manifested more clearly than in our positive discrimination in favour of beauty, and the growing body of research is uncovering even more advantages in having an attractive face, as if being attractive in the first place wasn't enough. Beauty may no longer be believed to suggest wisdom, but we do tend to equate it with many other positive attributes. It might seem unfair in this era of equality, but a raft of studies proves it: beauty is a lifelong advantage, because humans are predisposed to act well towards beautiful people. The ancient Greeks knew this and wished for their children to be born beautiful. In some countries, most notably Brazil, beauty can be used to change your life, a passport out of desperate circumstances, a step up in a rigidly stratified society. For middle-class Brazilians, looking attractive is so widely recognised as a benefit that plastic surgery is almost a rite of passage. Beauty has become a form of currency.

Can we define facial beauty?

Over the centuries, humans' assessment of beauty has changed. An obvious instance of this is the role of teeth in deciding a person's attractiveness. Before the development of dental science, missing teeth were so common that they were not a hindrance to being thought beautiful or handsome. In the nineteenth century British statesman Lord Palmerston was considered a handsome womaniser—'Lord Cupid', according to *The Times* in the 1830s—despite missing teeth. But regardless of changing tastes, there does seem to be some objective consensus about what constitutes facial beauty today.

Current research, when using computer graphics to isolate the characteristics that underlie our perception of beauty, found that averageness, symmetry and sexual dimorphism together constitute attractiveness. Each element was then varied in photographs and the reactions of viewers gauged to discover more about their roles and interplay. Interestingly, it seems that the same mix of the three elements produces an attractive face fairly consistently across all cultures. The researchers discovered that 'even with and between groups with little or no contact with Western standards of beauty, there is appreciable agreement in facial attractiveness ratings'. Children aged seven, twelve and seventeen have been found to rate beauty in the same way as adults, suggesting that there is a universality of perception that transcends not only different cultures but also different stages of human life.

A face that contains 'averageness' doesn't have any out-of-proportion features. Averageness was identified scientifically in the nineteenth century. In an 1870s experiment, British scientist Francis Galton (1822–1911), a half-cousin of Charles Darwin and an early pioneer of eugenics (a social philosophy that aimed to improve human genetic traits), collected pictures of male criminals and merged them together to form one composite image. He was trying to find a basic 'criminal face', expecting to find, using ideas from physiognomy, that criminals would share certain facial attributes that would make them identifiable and, presumably, not very attractive. However, instead of producing a criminal prototype that was ugly and malevolent looking, he kept ending up with attractive faces. He eventually realised that this was because the composite image evened out any strong features or irregularities, leaving him with an average face. At around the same time, Darwin received a letter from a correspondent who had noticed the same phenomenon: when two portraits were merged they always produced 'a decided improvement in beauty'. Averageness was confirmed as necessary in our perception of attractiveness in 2009, by researchers at the University of Texas. It has even been found that babies will gaze for longer at a photograph of a face derived from composite images than at one of a 'real' face.

It is possible that we find averageness attractive because it implies genetic fitness, something that we unconsciously look for when selecting a mate. Just like the diversity that formed Galton's composite image, an 'average' face is likely to have been formed from diverse genes, indicating strong immunity. Research at the University of Western Australia found that people with greater genetic diversity were rated the most attractive.

Symmetry, another key element of attractiveness identified, is the matching of the two sides of the face. It appears to be especially important in our perception of male attractiveness and masculinity. This may once again be linked to our unconscious search for good genes, as 'only high-quality individuals can maintain symmetric development under environmental and genetic stress'. It's possible, however, that we're hardwired to expect and accept a certain degree of visual asymmetry in a face, maybe due to the natural asymmetry that exists there. And, as William Hogarth rightly observed, too much regularity can tire the eye. He believed that humans prefer slight irregularity, such as that found in a three-legged stool or in a beautiful face in slight profile rather than seen front on.

The third element of beauty—sexual dimorphism—is evident in attributes that make a man's face masculine and a woman's feminine. In women this means rounded cheekbones on a face that is smaller along the jaw line but with fuller lips, while in men it means a heavier brow and jaw. Sexual dimorphism has been found to be more important than symmetry or averageness in our perception of facial attractiveness.

Hormones play a role in our liking of sexual dimorphism, with preference for sexually dimorphic features rising and falling along with our hormone levels. Ovulating women prefer more strongly masculine faces, but this preference decreases at other times of the month. Men with higher testosterone levels prefer women with more feminine faces. With its emphasis of sexual attributes such as healthy skin, full lips and clear eyes—which in earlier eras were all signs of being disease-free, fertile and healthy—sexual dimorphism may, like the other elements of attractiveness, be related to genetic selection of a mate.

However, women also have some preference for men with a slightly feminised face, rating them as being more cooperative and honest and as potentially making better parents. This suggests that when we look for a life partner, these sorts of traits may be seen as more useful than robust sexuality. In fact, 'feminisation, rather than sex exaggeration per se, is attractive in human faces'.

The role of proportion and variety

Humans like proportion; as the philosopher and theologian Thomas Aquinas noted in the thirteenth century, 'the senses delight in things duly proportioned'. Proportion has long been correlated with beauty. The golden ratio, also known as the divine proportion, has fascinated mathematicians for over two thousand years. It has been used by artists (either consciously or unconsciously) and occurs in the natural world—for example, in the proportions of shells and flowers. The geometrician Euclid of Alexandria defined the ratio in his work *Elements* in around 300 BCE:

> A straight line is said to have been cut in extreme
> and mean ratio when, as the whole line is to the
> greater segment, so is the greater to the lesser.

In other words, if a line is divided into two unequal sections, those sections are in the golden ratio if the ratio of the whole line to the larger section is the same as the ratio of the larger section to the smaller section.

For some reason—probably a correlation with some 'natural' pre-existing template in our brains—the golden ratio is pleasurable to humans, and we judge an object, be it a flower, a work of art or a human face, according to this proportion. The golden ratio can be found in many aspects of an attractive human face; this is what we mean when we say that a face is 'in proportion'.

Facial proportion has been an area of great interest over the centuries, and further rules have been suggested as to how the face should be proportioned in order to be attractive—for instance, that the width of the face should be two-thirds of its length, and that the length of the nose should be no greater than the distance between the eyes. A survey carried out in 2009 attempted to establish what people judge the most attractive facial proportions to be. Students were asked to rate a series of photographs of faces that had been digitally adjusted to vary the vertical and horizontal distances between features. The results indicated that the ideal distance between a woman's eyes and mouth is just over one-third of the overall length of her face from hairline to chin, while the optimal distance between a woman's pupils is a little under half of the width of her face from ear to ear.

These 'perfect' proportions actually correspond to the average face discussed earlier, which supports the research on the importance of averageness. However, when the researchers compared the ideal measurements to some well-known modern beauties, they didn't match. Angelina Jolie did not fit either the length or the width measurement, while Elizabeth Hurley fitted the measurement for length but not for width. Singer Shania Twain was found to have a perfect set of facial measurements. This perhaps indicates that, just as strict symmetry doesn't necessarily connote beauty, neither does strict proportion.

Symmetry in surgery

Symmetry is a real issue for plastic surgeons. It is unusual for a face to be perfectly symmetrical as it's constructed of two different sides that meet in the middle. In about 80 per cent of people, the right-hand side of the face is dominant. (This is unrelated to whether a person is right- or left-handed.) In fact, if a face is stronger on the left side rather than the right, we can feel that it looks strange without being able to say why. The differences are found in the facial skeleton, most significantly in the bony orbital cavity (around the eye), which projects less on the weaker side. This means the brow bone, the eye and the cheekbone are deeper set on that side and, as a consequence, the left brow is slightly lower because it is less supported by the bone. We tend to unconsciously focus on a face's dominant side—for instance, when looking at a newsreader on television. Asymmetry is usually not apparent in youth but shows increasingly with age.

Plastic surgery patients, not unreasonably, expect their surgeon to correct asymmetry in the course of surgery, but it's not that simple. If the surgeon brings both cheeks forwards to a symmetrical degree the result will exaggerate the original, naturally existing greater depth of the left eye. It requires aesthetic work to balance out some loss of symmetry at various levels so that even though the left cheek isn't as prominent as the right it doesn't look obviously different. The art is to *camouflage* the asymmetry without worsening it. It's a complex task.

Facial proportions are always in the background of assessment and surgical planning for plastic surgeons. They are useful guides for each individual face, templates against which the changes requested by patients can be made. This is particularly the case in surgery on the nose, as it helps to know the 'correct' proportion and appearance in order to enhance a person's overall attractiveness.

Variety can also be a source of attraction, in both the world in general and in the human face, as Hogarth noted. He wrote that 'the art of composing well is the art of varying well'. Variety in colour and form is what creates delight in a posy of flowers—a delight that fades when the flowers age and shrivel, losing their individual colours and shapes; there is pleasure to be found in winding walks, and in story plots that are hard to solve. Hogarth also observed that human hair can 'lead the eye a wanton kind of chase', thereby creating a 'delight' for our brain as well as our eyes, and that a face is more attractive when it is animated than when it is static. 'How soon does a face that wants expression, grow insipid, tho' it be ever so pretty?' Modern research agrees with his observation. When videos rather than photographs were used to assess attractiveness—allowing participants to see faces in action—more disagreement arose over which faces were attractive. Blinking, nodding and head tilting can all enhance a female face for a male observer. When meeting people, we find that someone talking or laughing can create attractiveness where before it may not have been apparent; on the other hand, the modern phenomenon of botox injections has created expressionless faces that are boring for those looking at them. In older people, there are definite benefits for attractiveness in movement: simply smiling can provide a 'temporary rejuvenation' by lighting up the face with expression.

Is appreciation of beauty hardwired?

Today we can see, using brain-scan technology, what an aesthetic experience looks like at the neurological level. Neuroaesthetics is the study of how our brain's wiring and appreciation of beauty intersect. It is a new science, only formally defined in 2002. We can now watch a brain while it's watching something else, which helps us to discover whether our responses are evolutionary—that is, if we're hardwired to like beauty.

When we look at beautiful artworks we undergo as much as a 10 per cent increase in blood flow to the medial orbitofrontal cortex, the part of the brain that is 'newer' in an evolutionary sense and responds to pleasure and reward processing. The amygdala, an 'older' part of the brain, which processes fear conditioning and rewards, is also activated. It is not unreasonable to take this finding a step further, from art to human beauty, and speculate that human beauty may also have this effect on us, since attractive people are good to look at and we feel better when we see them—the same response that we experience when looking at beautiful art. Babies are unformed assessors of the world around them, so it has been instructive to discover that, even when they're only two months old, they look for longer periods at attractive people. Conversely, our brains also respond with greater activity when we look at unattractive faces, raising the question that perhaps what we are really reacting to is a deviation from the norm.

The evidence seems conclusive that we are hardwired to appreciate beauty. No doubt this is about genes and survival. Researchers at the University of St Andrews have claimed that 'beauty increasingly appears to be ingrained in our biology: characteristics associated with evolutionary relevant advantages for choosing individuals [that are] perceived as attractive'. It would be interesting to know whether other species, especially our closest relative, the chimpanzee, also value visual attractiveness in a mate, and what elements would be combined in their definition of 'attractiveness'.

The advantages of being beautiful

Beautiful people are, on the whole, very well treated by those around them. It starts in infancy, when attractive babies are cooed over more than unattractive babies. In the playground, attractive children are more successful and are viewed by others as prestigious friends. They receive higher grades from their teachers and go on to acquire better jobs and to earn more money than their less attractive peers.

In 2011 US economist Daniel S Hamermesh coined the term 'pulchronomics'—the economics of beauty—to describe the measurable benefits of attractiveness. He calculated the economic advantage of beauty as being US$230,000 over the course of a lifetime, including people with jobs unrelated to appearance. In his 1999 research into facial awareness, Randy Thornhill, distinguished professor at the University of New Mexico's Department of Biology, found that 'the prediction that attractive people of all ages receive favourable treatment from others is upheld by the available evidence'. Beauty can even be a predictor of health in the later stages of life.

The way in which we view ourselves has been shown to affect our attractiveness. Those who believe themselves to be attractive and of 'high mate value' are more likely to attract and retain a 'high-value' mate, possibly accounting for the frequent phenomenon of attractive people partnering with other attractive people. Research by the London School of Economics published in *The Australian* in January 2011 found that children of attractive people are not only more likely to be attractive than the norm but also more intelligent, with IQs up to fourteen points higher than average. And, as if that's not enough, *The Age* reported in April 2011 that researchers at the University of

Texas had found beautiful people to be happier—their happiness largely the result of the economic advantages their beauty had bestowed on them.

This sort of research is rarely well received: the observation that beauty has advantages is not popular. We feel some contempt for the notion that we judge people on their looks alone. Nobody wants to know that mating success, earning potential, happiness and longevity are all positively correlated with attractiveness. What does it say about the society we live in? The idea also raises fears, for if beauty is truly such an advantage and we now have the surgical means to make anyone beautiful, where does that leave us?

Academic discussions about the benefits of beauty and the disadvantages of being unattractive are developing. In *The Beauty Bias* (2010), Stanford Law School professor Deborah Rhode claimed that beauty should not be allowed to pay, that women's obsession with looks and fashion is detrimental to themselves and to society, and that the whole issue of 'appearance discrimination' in employment should be addressed by the state. She had good reason to argue this case. Research into pulchronomics has found that unattractive women earn 3 per cent less than average-looking women and that unattractive men earn 22 per cent less than their average-looking counterparts. Even quarterbacks are affected: unattractive quarterbacks earn 12 per cent less than better-looking quarterbacks. Rhode believes that in time unattractive people may receive official protection from the government of the sort that currently protects the rights of people with disabilities in developed countries.

Appearance discrimination is a burgeoning issue, but it's not new. The social and economic significance of appearance was noticed by early-modern plastic surgeons, including the French doctor Suzanne Noël (1878–1954). Some of her patients in the 1920s were unable to afford to eat because they could not find work; one even fainted from hunger in her surgery. These patients visited Noël not out of vanity but because of the need to look attractive enough to be employable. After surgery they tended to find work, an effect that so interested Noël that she wrote a book about it: *Aesthetic Surgery and Its Social Significance* (1926).

Perhaps, as Naomi Wolf wrote in *The Beauty Myth* (1991), beauty is a form of currency, though in a different way from that which pulchronomics describes. Wolf argued that our obsession with beauty is a political tool used against women to destabilise their achievements. She thought that as women have gained power in areas traditionally occupied by men, men have responded by creating a new form of currency for women: beauty. This has forced women to compete on a new playing field, explaining why the rise of women's power since the 1980s has corresponded with many women feeling worse about themselves rather than better. They have increased anxiety about their appearance, a growing obsession with their physicality, a terror of ageing and an increasing fixation on ideals of female beauty.

Recently, the reverse of this idea has also received attention—the notion of women owning 'erotic capital', their attractiveness being a form of currency that can be used to their advantage. Unlike economic or social capital, this is not limited by what level of society a woman is born into: she can use what she has in the way of looks to reach where she wants to go. The obvious downside to this is that naturally beautiful people can end up using their looks at the expense of developing proper life skills, making the privileged life that beauty brings a workable option only until the beauty fades or is lost.

Beauty is a source of delight. Humans are profoundly affected by it, moved to create songs and poetry, as well as to do battle and to take vengeance in its name. The ancient Greeks wrote extensively about beauty; for Plato this was a joyful recognition of the human in its perfect form, remembered by our souls from the time we spent with the gods. The ancient philosopher Plotinus similarly believed that we respond to physical beauty because in it 'we dimly recognise its paradigm', the perfect form. He claimed that the source of all beautiful things is the Good, which is also the source of their beauty.

It's quite clear that people with attractive or beautiful faces have a head start in most aspects of their lives. It's interesting that the benefits are bestowed on them by other people, often acting quite unconsciously, in a variety of ways. In addition, there must also be a subconscious power that comes from being treated better by other people—it's certainly a compelling argument in favour of having an attractive face.

5

The wrong face

*People of normal appearance can seldom imagine
the tragic inner feelings which pervade, poison and
dominate the lives of less fortunate people, ever
conscious of a facial deformity or abnormality.*

Charles Willi

What does it feel like to have a face that isn't right, a face that you are constantly aware of and—just in case you do forget it for a moment—are reminded of by other people's reactions to it? Those of us with a 'normal' face can gain an inkling of what this is like when we go out in public with a bloodshot eye, a blemish or a cold sore. Feeling self-conscious is bad enough, but it is made worse when we see people's eyes quickly travel to the area we most hope they won't notice, after which there is a second or two of adjustment while they try not to stare and we both try to overcome the moment and 'act normally'. A bloodshot eye leaves us feeling temporarily embarrassed and maybe a bit disappointed that the social encounter had to take place while we looked as we did. But for people who live with permanent facial irregularity—even something as apparently simple as a scar, sagging eyelids or a large nose—life is altered because of it.

Civil inattention

Author Laura Greenwald has recorded a person with facial difference commenting that

> [we] wear our imperfections like labels on our faces every day, all the time—in photos, at formal events, interviewing for a job and meeting someone for the first time.

One of the main problems for these people is the loss of a little noticed but essential attribute called 'civil inattention', described by Frances Cooke MacGregor as being the attribute that allows us to move anonymously and unnoticed in public places without thinking overly about ourselves. Rosemarie Garland-Thomson, an expert in disability studies, has confirmed the importance of this, writing that many of us forget that 'one of the privileges of normalcy in modernity is not being noticeable, not being stared at, not being seen'. With facial disfigurement, this ability to move about unnoticed is replaced by second looks, intrusive glances, stares, whispers, avoidance and, in the worst extremes, attack.

Being stared at is something we humans find very difficult. It makes us too aware of ourselves, creating an atmosphere of apprehension and threat that makes it hard to behave normally. This is probably a primeval response from the days when to be stared at meant we were being singled out from the group as a potential meal. In the primate world staring is used to exert power, and the object animal has two options: to stare back and signal defiance or to look away and signal submission. Every day in the park our dogs do something similar, with the lowest in the pack avoiding eye contact when things get difficult. As Darwin noted, a stare can be so powerful that it alone is enough to make the target blush without any other form of contact. Even when the stare is only believed to have been given, it still undermines a person's confidence. Patients frequently tell me that when they sit in their car in traffic, they'll put up their hand to cover the part of their face they feel self-conscious about—typically a prominent nose—so other motorists don't look over and see it. I actually ask prospective patients about what they do at a red light, as a form of screening test, because I have found those who describe doing this are usually good candidates for surgery.

A burdensome face

Ian was a tall young man who walked into my consulting room with his face down, his head encased in a woollen beanie, followed quietly by his mother. I took one look at his downcast demeanour and decided that I wasn't going to operate. There seemed to be something wrong and he didn't present as a good candidate for surgery. Respectfully I listened to his story and as it unfolded my opinion of him began to change.

When Ian was ten years old he had been diagnosed with Tourette's syndrome, a neurological condition characterised by uncontrolled twitches and grimacing and often accompanied by a loud involuntary vocal component. Within six months of diagnosis he had gained thirty kilograms, from the medication and from his use of food as an emotional outlet. As a teenager he had been bullied, which left him feeling worthless and crying himself to sleep each night. Following his adolescence he outgrew the symptoms of Tourette's, but the weight remained. Between the ages of eighteen and twenty, he lost ninety kilograms through diet, exercise and impressive willpower. But even then his problems weren't over. The loss of weight created a new problem, visible on his face: he had loose, droopy skin over his jaw and neck, and his neck continued without definition from the tip of his chin to his chest. His face appeared to have dropped, and his eyes looked sunken, an effect exacerbated by his naturally flat cheekbones.

Just as the research we looked at would have predicted, his appearance had led to feelings of shame and a diminished social life, as Ian chose to stay at home rather than risk social encounters. He described his looks as a 'burden': a reflection of the journey he'd taken through life and not a reflection of who he was.

> There was not a day that I would leave home without covering my head with a hat or hooded sweater, something to guard me from public embarrassment. I didn't feel I could assimilate, especially in a society so intensely driven by body image.

As it turned out, my reaction to Ian when he walked into my consulting room was a classic instance of incorrectly judging a person by their facial appearance—the very reason he had come to seek my help.

Facial irregularity is front and centre in every interaction: unlike other problems, it can't be revealed to others only when the sufferer is ready to do so. Over time, many people with a facial irregularity or heightened facial awareness experience feelings of shame related to their appearance and, as a result, choose to hide themselves away. This may sound extreme, but it has been confirmed by three decades of research. Christine Pitt, founder of Let's Face It, an organisation based in the United Kingdom that puts people with a facial disfigurement in touch with others in the same situation, believes that more than half of the people who have a facial difference simply take themselves away from society.

Honoré de Balzac

Nineteenth-century French playwright and novelist Honoré de Balzac had a face that didn't reflect his inner soul, but was fortunate to live in an era when this did not have to be revealed to his readers. When he was pushed to have his portrait painted at the age of thirty-seven, he lamented the disillusion it would create when his female readers saw his face. He realised his appearance, when made public, would not match the expectations of those female readers who felt they knew him from his words. With his big head, bulbous nose, double chin and generally unattractive appearance, he did not look as they might have expected a great and revered writer to look. Some radio broadcasters must have felt the same when television was introduced—not all made the transition to the new visual medium.

Balzac might have been consoled by Plotinus. When asked by his students to have his portrait painted, the ancient philosopher replied that his face wasn't him at all, merely his husk. To have a portrait painted would therefore be creating a husk of a husk, an illusion quite unable to convey the most important thing—his soul. The face may be only our surface, but it's the surface of the 'self', the surface that matters. (In the end, Plotinus did have his portrait painted.)

Minotaur syndrome

A large amount of aesthetic plastic surgery is triggered by the immense suffering that people endure when their face doesn't match their personality. In 1993, plastic surgeon Paolo G Morselli coined the term 'Minotaur syndrome' to describe the discrepancy between a person's facial appearance and their inner personality, and the suffering caused when they are incorrectly judged by others. In Greek mythology, the Minotaur was a monster with the body of a human but the head of a bull. People suffering from this syndrome become victims of their looks.

A middle-aged male patient of mine was a classic example of the Minotaur syndrome. His face was dominated by thick, downcast eyebrows; classic 'Mephistopheles eyebrows', named after the mythical medieval devil. The actor Jack Nicholson uses his similarly shaped eyebrows to dramatic effect, giving a demonic look to some of the character roles he plays. For my patient, the effect was to make him look perpetually angry, in fact quite frightening. People would naturally feel wary of him, even though they had no reason to. It's not difficult to see how this mismatch would have affected his life. The Minotaur syndrome can also apply to another, larger group in society: those undergoing facial ageing. Many people who see the changes of ageing on their face but still feel youthful inside find this mismatch is a cause of considerable distress and loss of confidence. It's one of the often overlooked but profound psychological effects of facial ageing.

Behind the face

Maxwell Maltz (1899–1975), famous for his classic motivational self-help book *Psycho-Cybernetics* (1960), was actually a plastic surgeon. While he was one of the first to recognise the power of facial surgery to change a person's life for the better, he also developed theories of human motivation and behaviour through his observations of the surprising disconnect between some outcomes of plastic surgery and patient satisfaction or dissatisfaction. He became fascinated by the fact that while most people experienced an almost immediate rise in self-esteem, others, no matter how good their surgery, simply transferred their dissatisfaction to another area and their emotional stress remained unaltered. They contined to act as if the facial problem still existed. Maltz began to realise that to achieve a success-ful outcome the patient needed to align their self-image along with their changed face. They needed to see themselves differ-ently, otherwise the psychological problem remained. For some patients this was not possible, due to deeper psychological impediments. In some instances the change of face unwittingly led to other problems arising from tampering with their self-image. For instance, Maltz operated on a German boy who had a scar on his face, only to find that the boy suffered depression as a result. It turned out that the boy had thought of himself as a warrior, and his sense of identity had been altered once his scar was no longer so noticeable.

Maltz realised that the way we see ourselves is the basis for our behaviour, and that some of us have distorted perceptions of self, in which instance surgery is not the answer. He urged surgeons to learn about each patient and to look for unrealistic expectations—that is, to address the psychological needs as well as the physical needs of patients.

At this point in our discussion it is important to make a distinction between those people who are unhappy with their facial or bodily appearance because of an existing irregularity or disfigurement discernible to others, and those people who have an illness—body dysmorphic disorder—due to which they develop a 'distressing or impaired preoccupation with a non-existent or minimal appearance flaw'. The condition has also been known as 'body hypochondria' or 'the insatiable patient'. Sufferers are convinced that some aspect of their appearance is unattractive, deformed, ugly or 'not right', even though to others the flaw seems not to exist or to be a minor blemish. The face is a frequent site for this attention, especially the hair, nose and skin.

Body dysmorphic disorder can seem a perplexing condition, but we do have an idea of the way in which it develops. Researcher Beverley McNamara has described it in an interesting way: 'Each human being has two bodies: an individual body acquired at birth and the social body acquired through socialisation'. The social body is the result of sensory input about us, which is influenced by emotional factors such as personal desires and attitudes, and interactions with others (parents telling their child that he's fat, for instance). As a result, our perception of our body or face is more an abstract idea than a true reflection of the reality. This is how people with body dysmorphic disorder can look in the mirror and see something quite different from their actual reflection.

Although only 2 per cent of the population is affected, plastic surgeons see a large number of body dysmorphic disorder sufferers, estimated to be up to 15 per cent of patients, as surgery is understandably seen by them to be a solution to their problems. Sufferers often mask their condition in their desperation for surgery, but surgery is very rarely the answer, even if it is deemed that an improvement can be made to a certain feature. Wooing the surgeon by flattery, to get their agreement, is a typical ploy: 'I've been to the other surgeons but you're the best,' or 'You did a great job, but I'd be happy if you did a little bit more'. No matter how good the result, the patient will remain focused on the same problem or turn to another 'problem area'.

In some instances surgery simply exacerbates negative feelings about the perceived problem, contrary to the reaction of most patients, whose body image improves post-operatively.

Obviously, this disorder and others like it can lead to a person receiving numerous operations, either from unscrupulous practitioners or from practitioners who don't recognise the psychological symptoms. It is the surgeon's responsibility to find patients' real motivations, especially with body dysmorphic disorder sufferers, and to ensure that those patients don't enter an unnecessary or unhelpful series of surgical procedures.

Beautiful stranger

In her book *Beautiful Stranger*, Hope Donahue provided a tragic insight into what can happen when someone is given the surgery they request, but whose real problem exists beyond the realm of surgery. Donahue was a naturally beautiful young woman who underwent multiple surgical procedures—seven before the age of twenty-seven—in the belief that if she could perfect her appearance she could overcome her unhappiness. Much later she realised that her appearance anxiety was more to do with psychological issues arising from having grown up surrounded by wealth and material comforts yet devoid of the family values and support that most of us associate with good thinking and a satisfying life. The physical ordeal of surgery allowed her to avoid the reality. To help fill the vacuum she fantasised that her surgeon would fall in love with her, hoping that out of nothing something might arise. Her words show that the help she needed would never be provided by surgery.

> It wasn't long before my visits to his office were what I
> lived for. I needed them to provide me the human contact,
> excitement, the fulfilment I wasn't getting anywhere else
> in my life.

As she approached surgery she would think:

> I want to be able to look in the mirror and not see only
> what I think is wrong and unattractive. I want to be loved.
> Can you do all that, doctor?

The human face is so central to human life that its importance is not just limited to our personal perceptions of ourselves; it's also social and even political. To live behind the 'wrong face' is to exist but in a diminished way, your life dictated by your features.

It can be a problem as apparently simple as the 'wrong' eyebrows or some other dominating feature. The looks that others bestow on us are a powerful factor in our ability to live in society and our potential for happiness.

6

Facial ageing

The great secret that all old people share is that you
really haven't changed in seventy or eighty years.
Your body changes, but you don't change at all.
And that, of course, causes great confusion.

Doris Lessing

We are surrounded by more older people in the twenty-first century than in any previous era. In 1950, globally, one in every twenty people was sixty-five years old or more. In 2000 the figure was one in every fourteen, and it has been predicted that by 2050 it will be almost one in every six. According to the United Nations, this growth in worldwide population ageing is unprecedented, without parallel in human history, and is set to endure. In Australia, the life expectancy of a man born at the start of the twentieth century was fifty-five; for a man born in 2006 it was seventy-nine.

The corresponding figures for women were fifty-nine and eighty-three, respectively. These are astonishing figures, and a key element has been the reduction in mortality rates in people over fifty, especially since 1970. This means that the increase in life expectancy is not being driven by lower infant mortality; we really are living longer.

And as we live longer, we don't see older people as being 'old'. The whole notion of age has been recast: it's commonly said that the age of fifty, instead of being a time of maturity and slowing down, has become 'the new forty', for many people one of their busiest decades. And so it goes on through each decade. We work, socialise and maintain a vital role in the world long past the age at which our parents decided to start taking it easy. And because we're fit, active and expect to live longer, we also expect our external appearance to match how we're feeling in the decades of middle age and beyond.

Looking your age

Facial ageing is a result of the phenomenon of living longer. Medical science has made enormous strides in treating disease and infection—so people generally don't die at as young an age as they did in the past—but the actual signs of age have so far been unaffected by medical advances. Simply because people are alive for longer they look old for longer. The ageing process is not linear but exponential, meaning that the rate of visible ageing increases each year. The average sixty-year-old tends to look a great deal older than the average fifty-year-old, with most of the change happening in the final few years of the decade. That's why people frequently comment that they seemed to 'age overnight'.

Most people are not prepared for these facial changes, and the psychological impact can be profound. For some, the loss of confidence that accompanies facial ageing is damaging to a degree they could never have believed when they were younger. The changes start well before we even begin to feel old, and for a lot of people the first awareness of their ageing appearance comes when they occasionally look tired even though they don't feel tired. That gradually increases to looking tired for a few days each week, until they discover that they are looking tired on most days. That look of tiredness, so often used to describe facial ageing, has in fact become their new face. People often notice themselves—almost as if seeing an ageing stranger—in a window reflection or a changing room mirror and feel shocked by what they see. It's as though a mask has suddenly appeared, obscuring the face they have known all their life. Although the 'mask of ageing' is the most commonly used expression, some people also describe their ageing face as looking 'untidy' or 'dissolute', which, particularly for those who dislike untidiness and take pride in the way they dress and appear in public, can be distressing. At this point, many people begin to feel less certain that facial ageing can be shrugged off as irrelevant.

Until people experience ageing for themselves, they don't realise how bewildering it can be to have your face change so quickly. Suddenly (or so it seems) a middle-aged person can find themselves scarcely able to reconcile the person they know themselves to be with the person they see in the mirror. Mostly, people liked the face that has now become obscured with ageing, and its loss forms part of the grieving that can accompany the loss of youth. Even those who don't lament this loss can find they lament the loss of a face that told people more about them than just their age. They start to notice that people speak to them differently, even though they don't feel different. The dismay caused by ageing is so common and so strongly experienced by older people that it almost forms a 'psychology of facial ageing'. Adding to the frustration is the discovery that the process can't be mitigated by exercise, skin creams or inner peace. Older people are forced to wear their new look without any control or consent.

It can be frightening to no longer look like the person you've always been. Middle-aged and older people have to contend with a vast disparity between who they feel they are and what they look like to others. The mismatch can lead to despondency and loss of confidence. Just as people with facial abnormalities struggle with the judgements of others, so people with facial ageing struggle, especially with comments suggesting they look tired, unwell, irritable or out of touch. Understandably, they resent such comments. They want to be addressed as the person they are, rather than the person they look like.

Invisible age

Commonly, people—especially women—begin to feel 'invisible' once they reach a certain age, as if they have almost ceased to exist as far as the wider world is concerned. This may be because young women are, in general, more noticed than young men, so when that attention fades they are more aware of it. One of my patients, a teacher, actually performed a little test on this. One day she took a group of students to a shopping centre and left them for a few moments while, out of sight, she put on a grey wig to give her the appearance of an older woman. She then returned and walked past the students. They didn't recognise her. They didn't even *look at* her.

Ageing gracefully?

'Ageing gracefully' is a reassuring phrase which suggests that as we age we garner grace and wisdom, and that these experiences show on our faces. Karen DeCrow, a former president of the US National Organization for Women, wrote for *The New York Times* in September 1990 that 'if there is anything behind a face, that face improves with age. Lines show distinction and character; they show that someone has lived; that one may know something'. We probably all hope that we will develop in grace and wisdom as we age and that our character will both mellow and deepen. That is how we would like it to be, how we think it *should* be as we age. But it is rarely the case that such attributes show on the face. Sadly, as a quick glance around any street will prove, most people simply don't age gracefully.

People who talk about ageing gracefully tend to be younger, and it is hard when you're young to understand the sadness that comes with ageing. When young people look tired, it's usually because they are. They don't have to live with that look every day. The idea of ageing gracefully is described in the following text written by author Naomi Wolf, which provides an attractive but idealised description of what facial ageing should be.

> If a woman is healthy she lives to grow old; as she thrives, she reacts and speaks and shows emotion, and grows into her face. Lines trace her thought and radiate from the corners of her eyes after decades of laughter, closing together like fans as she smiles.

Wolf then describes forehead lines as 'horizontal creases of surprise, delight, compassion and good talk', while the creases around the mouth demonstrate 'a lifetime of kissing or speaking and weeping'. The loose skin around the face and throat show sensual dignity. The total effect of facial ageing, according to Wolf, is to strengthen the facial features, directly reflecting the strengthening of personality that comes with age.

. If this were a realistic description of facial ageing, most of us would happily accept it. We would enjoy the thought that our face becomes more 'me' than it was in youth. If facial ageing were simply a matter of a few character lines around the eyes or mouth, as Wolf suggested, rejuvenation surgery would never have become the specialty that it has. But in reality, people's distress isn't the result of a few 'character lines' at all. It comes from appearing to themselves and others as someone quite different from how they feel inside. It's about the loss of a face they liked and, most especially, it's about the downcast and inescapable look of tiredness that accompanies middle age. It's also about the loss of a sense of self. For many, all these changes will create their first experience of facial awareness and lead to a loss of confidence in their daily interactions and social relationships, just as they are moving into a new stage of life.

The real me

Mary was a country woman of about seventy who had an aged face and profound hooding over her eyes. She was referred to me by her GP in the country because the hooding was affecting her vision, which is not uncommon when it becomes so advanced. Her 'mask of ageing' was so severe that her face resembled a wall of skin through which her eyes were barely visible.

When I told her that the standard, simple treatment for this sort of eyelid problem was quite different to a proper blepharoplasty performed for aesthetic reasons, she chose to have a blepharoplasty—and later went on to have a face lift.

She explained: 'I was a typical woman. I used to love to go shopping and I was also secretary of the bowls club. But I became so despondent about my appearance—I would go into a shop and there would be these young girls serving and I could see them thinking, "Why is that old bag looking at these fashionable clothes ... as if clothes would make any difference!" I became so depressed I even gave up being secretary of the bowls club.'

After her surgery, when I told her she looked like a different person, she rebuked me, with words that explain exactly the way many people feel about facial ageing. 'No I don't,' she said firmly. 'This *is* the real me. That other person wasn't.'

7

Changing face

It is difficult ... to escape becoming the person
which others believe one to be. A slave is twice
enslaved, once by his chains and once again
by the glances that fall upon him and say
'thou slave.'

Thornton Wilder

The decision to have facial surgery is a major one and is made after great consideration, but if it lightens a burden and creates the ability to live life more confidently, then the trade-off is well worth while. In a later chapter we look more closely at patient motivation, but the patients quoted here tell their stories of what it's like live with facial awareness and how it feels to be relieved of the burden by surgery.

I look in the mirror and like what I see

All I ever wanted to be was plain and unremarkable. When I entered secondary school in 1975, at twelve years old, it was the age of the blonde surfie chick, the Big M girls and Farrah Fawcett. Like many, I didn't fit the mould. But I suffered more than most as I had recently returned from living overseas and so didn't fit in, and I was afflicted with a flat 'punched-in' face, oversized chin, red hair, freckles, glasses and too many brains. For years I had been teased about what I looked like but it did not get vicious until my fifteenth and sixteenth years, which were the worst.

I started to pile on makeup in an attempt to compensate for my inadequacies. I developed the habit of comfort eating, bingeing followed by dieting. I also learnt that avoiding eye contact helped to discourage the attention of bullies. I cultivated the habit of walking with eyes downcast, and withdrew into my head.

Throughout my university years and my twenties the only relationships I had with men involved just friendship or just sex—no boyfriends and never any dates—while all around me people were dating and getting married. When I was nearly thirty I stumbled across a self-development course that made me confront my low self-esteem. After much work a great weight lifted and I realised that I had a choice. I could accept what I looked like—or get it changed. I then made my decision to investigate plastic surgery.

I asked others what they thought. People who cared about me told me there was nothing wrong with me, which confused me endlessly as it totally contradicted the feedback I had received from the rest of the world for years. Two friends, however, had the courage to tell me that I would look better with the surgery I was considering. 'I used to notice it and although I don't notice anymore, you would definitely look better if you had it fixed,' said one. This meant a lot to me.

Today, many years [after surgery], I look in the mirror and like what I see. I no longer recoil when I see myself in a photograph. I no longer automatically assume that any rejection by men is a result of what I look like. Nowadays I look like the majority of the population, not perfect but perfectly acceptable. I have achieved my goal of being unremarkable. In recent years an admirer told me, 'The nicest thing about you is that you don't know you are attractive.'

Those of us who are born with the wrong ticket in the aesthetic genetic lottery suffer twice. First we are judged by those who find us visually lacking. Then, when we do something about it, we are judged again. Judged by the very people who are born with proportionate faces and bodies, who see no contradiction when they straighten their teeth, colour their hair and wear contact lenses, makeup and brassieres. I say to the critics: it took great misery, and then great courage and expense, for me to finally take the plunge and have cosmetic plastic surgery to redress disproportionate facial features and become unremarkable like the majority of the population. In this process I have had to deal with yet another wave of judgement for the injustice people like me have suffered. Cosmetic plastic surgery is a band-aid. If you can stop human beings from being aesthetically discriminating then you will have the cure.

Aesthetic and rejuvenation surgery

A young man whose face had been badly affected by significant weight loss described being acutely aware of the burden of his facial appearance: 'I felt looked at, as though people were saying, "Don't sit next to him"'. After undergoing facial aesthetic surgery he found immense relief to be once more a subject of civil inattention. 'It's so wonderful to not be noticed,' he said, 'to just glide in like anyone else'.

New beginnings

I think I started to notice the difference in my looks in high school. I was constantly aware of my neck and the fact that it was different to everyone else's. I never liked photos of myself unless they were taken from above where you couldn't see it. I would play with my earrings when I crossed the street so that people in cars couldn't see my face and I developed a habit of speaking with my hands near my mouth to try and hide it. I had what doctors termed a 'thickness of the neck': excess fatty tissue that was like a large double chin and made me look bigger than I was. Doctors would comment and ask if I'd had thyroid checks. Whenever the subject was brought up I would immediately put my hands under my chin to try and hide it. It was such a sensitive subject.

People have asked me if I was scared or had second thoughts before my surgery. I can confidently say no. This wasn't a 'spur of the moment' decision for me. I didn't do this to look like an airbrushed model on the front cover of a magazine. It was just something I knew I had to do for myself, to give myself a chance to finally be comfortable in my own skin. From the moment I chose to go ahead with the surgery, I have had nothing but support and positive comments from everyone. They all stood by my decision and helped me through my recovery.

I am over the moon with my result. On my fifth-week appointment I was shown my photos that were taken before the operation. The tears welled up and I could hardly look at them. My confidence has grown gradually. I don't hide my face as much and I can have my photo taken without dreading what I look like. But I am now ready for a new beginning.

Patients seek rejuvenation surgery to find a balance between feeling relatively youthful while the ageing process continues unabated. The desire to remain looking vigorous and not capitulate to ageing isn't new. The surgeon Mario González-Ulloa, who researched the history of facial rejuvenation during the twentieth century, noted

> the constant, and constantly powerful, motive of vital men and women of every era to keep their facial and bodily appearance in youthful harmony with their inner feelings of strength and their vigour in action.

It seems to me to be a very natural and understandable motive, and never more so than in the twenty-first century when we can expect to live healthier and longer lives than ever before.

Facial ageing can also cause workplace insecurity. People can appear to be too old to cope with new technology or simply irrelevant to contemporary ways of doing things. Many of the earliest face lift patients, at the start of the twentieth century, turned to surgery as a means of staying in work, so this is a problem that preceded the arrival of today's technology. Professor Emil Meirowsky wrote in 1931 that

> the bitter struggle for existence compels each individual to take care that he is not cast aside too early as 'old iron' and expelled from the fight for bread and board.

However, throughout the history of facial rejuvenation it has aroused unease, especially the face lift. For some it's almost akin to cheating; for others it's a sign of society gone mad for youth, fed by the 'questionable' values of celebrities, sportspeople and politicians.

Premature ageing

I couldn't hide what my face had started to show; with all the stress and misery [from depression following a break-up] I had aged prematurely. I looked ten years older, my face was thin, my skin had sagged, my eyes were sunken in, and I had jowls. I was only thirty-nine. My friends, family and colleagues had started to become concerned, commenting that I looked too thin in the face, and that was them being polite. I felt even more miserable every time I looked in the mirror. I saw an old lady staring back at me. I lost all confidence and only left the house to go to work.

The results [of facial surgery] have been amazing, so natural-looking. I have my confidence back. I am living again. I am dating. I love being me again.

Contrary to commonly held belief, rejuvenation patients do not refuse to admit to ageing or hope that their surgery will miraculously turn the clock back to their youth. Rather, they seek to remove the mask and have their real face back again. They are normally healthy people involved in the world and, indeed, often at the peak of their activity.

Having spent their life not giving a lot of thought to their looks, the patient is suddenly confronted with the reality of how important their face is and its vital role in their sense of identity. Before undergoing facial rejuvenation they often have to re-evaluate their beliefs about plastic surgery, the superficiality of appearances or youthful convictions that they would age with equanimity. These are easy opinions to hold in youth, when our ideas about ageing are an abstract set of notions about a future that seems a long way off. At that point we assume that middle-aged or older people feel their age and don't mind looking like they do. In reality, this is rarely the case.

It may appear that rejuvenation patients form a separate group, motivated by different concerns, from those who seek surgery to correct or improve the appearance of an actual abnormality. But the motivation is essentially similar: they want to live their lives more joyously, freed of a deforming or obscuring feature that has negatively affected their life. A woman in her seventies who had had several procedures since her mid-fifties expressed her delight about not looking her age: 'I feel younger. I act younger. The interesting thing is that people of all ages and occupations treat me differently because they think I am younger. I love it!'

Comfortable in my own skin

I was the fat kid with acne at school, known as Pizza Face even before puberty. The first time I considered surgery on my face I was sixteen. I was staring in the mirror at my ravaged skin, where acne of all forms and shapes had taken residence from scalp to breast. I seriously considered getting a knife from the kitchen and cutting sections of my face off—it just seemed the only way I could look 'normal'. In my twenties a heavy-duty acne drug did end the acne life cycle, but I was left with extensive scarring, especially on my face. I always looked at the moon with fondness: my brother in damaged surfaces!

When I decided to have a face lift, it was only ever about reducing the scarring. I entered that room knowing exactly what I was doing and why. I strongly believe that surgery for aesthetic reasons is a valuable tool for psychological healing. Now, my face is not pockmark free, but that would have been a fantasy, never the goal. I'm a practical woman. What's important is that my face is perfect, for me.

Three times in the last twelve months I've had men tell me that I'm beautiful. In my life I don't recall anyone but my mother saying that, and she was just trying to boost my confidence. I acknowledge that psychological damage from a lifetime of social rejection, bad skin and weight problems left a toll that I'm still dealing with, but I genuinely believe those men called me beautiful because I'm now comfortable in my own skin. The surgery changed my life; afterwards I quickly reached my goal weight and at forty-four I'm the fittest I've ever been in my life. I'm grateful and happy that through surgery I've made the best of what God gave me.

When faces aren't right, people suffer. Whatever the cause—disfigurement, accident, genes, ageing or the perception of the face's owner—it is indisputable that right from the start demand for aesthetic plastic surgery arose from deep psychological distress related to the face, and not from issues of vanity—as it continues to be today. When we look to the origins of aesthetic plastic surgery, which stretch back to antiquity, we find countless people enduring unbelievable pain, the potential for death from infection and great suffering, just to achieve facial normality. Even though it wasn't until the late nineteenth century that anaesthesia and antisepsis became available, these people still chose to have surgery rather than suffer the psychological distress of living behind a face that wasn't right.

Working rejuvenation

I worked with adolescents and as I was growing older the gap between me and them was growing and they were now talking about me as being their mother, so it was harder for me to relate to the population I was working with. I wanted to be able to bridge that gap a bit: it was a professional reason as much as a personal [one]—I wanted to be who I was exactly but looking a bit younger.

Now I'm really happy. I definitely notice people look at me more, they interact with me more, they engage with me more. And I don't think it's just that I engage them. Without a shadow of a doubt, younger people talk to me more, they'll come and chat to me where they never did that before.

Part 2

The development of aesthetic plastic surgery

In all human relationships, it is the face that is the symbol of or synonymous with the person, the region where the sense of self is located ... the focus of attention whenever people meet.

Frances C Macgregor

8

The Indian method

A man without a nose [arouses] horror and
loathing and people are apt to regard the deformity
as a just punishment for his sins … No one ever asks
whether the nose was lost because a beam fell on it,
or whether it was destroyed by scrofula or syphilis.

John Friedrich Dieffenbach

Few who saw the cover of *Time* magazine in August 2010 could forget the image: a photograph of a beautiful young girl with two gaping holes in the centre of her face where the tip of her nose had been removed. Those who saw it were left in no doubt about the cruelty of facial disfigurement.

For millennia, facial mutilation has been used as punishment or vengeance against enemies, and as a way of defining and owning people. The Romans tattooed their slaves between the eyes, in the manner of farmers branding cattle, while in countries such as Burma and Japan criminals were tattooed on their face so they were clearly marked out within society. Rhinokopia, or removal of the nose tip, as suffered by the young girl on the cover of *Time*, was first recorded as a punishment in ancient India, where it was exacted on criminals. At various times it has also been used against political enemies and to punish conquered communities. It was also practised in Byzantine Europe: Emperor Justinian II was known as Rhinotmetus, or 'one with an amputated nose', as a result of rhinokopia inflicted on him by his enemies following his deposition. This mutilation would have made him ineligible to rule; however, he did succeed in becoming emperor for a second time—allegedly by wearing a gold nasal prosthesis—before eventually being beheaded. Sadly, as demonstrated by *Time*, rhinokopia continues today in parts of the world. It endures because it is a disturbingly perfect act of aggression, condemning victims not to death itself but to a living death, forcing them to see out their lives as hideous outcasts, repellent to themselves, their family and their society. From the moment of disfigurement, every waking hour of that person revolves around that simple act. It's a psychological assault effected by physical means, and it is hard to think of any other act that could so ruin a life.

The same thinking lies behind other facial mutilations, such as the current spate of acid attacks on women in Colombia, where the perpetrator uses the woman's face as a site of vengeance. One hundred and fifty acid attacks took place in 2011, and a hundred had already been recorded within the first five months of 2012. Such acts occur throughout the world, often carried out by an ex-lover whose desire to punish the victim leads to a sadistically planned assault; he wants the woman to live but to have her life reduced to a reminder of his rage. He will control and humiliate the victim until she dies. *The Washington Post* reported in August 2012 that a man who had paid a child $1.75 to drench his former lover in acid told his victim, 'If you're not mine, then no one will have you'. Another victim, a previously attractive woman who now wears an elastic mask, breathes through a tube and has been reduced to begging for food, described herself as looking like a monster. 'Life is too hard and I'm alone,' she said. One woman, who ended up enduring fifty surgeries over nine years, had acid thrown in her face by a stranger who shouted, 'This is so you don't think you're so pretty'. The photographer who took the women's pictures for *The Washington Post* found himself disturbed by the experience, feeling that hiding behind a camera was not an appropriate response.

Nose-cut Town

In around 1770 the city of Kirtipoor in Nepal was the scene of a mass rhinokopia for which we have the eyewitness account of a Catholic priest called Father Giuseppe, recorded in the Asiatic Society's periodical *Asiatick Researches*. Following the surrender of the inhabitants to the Gurkha army after a long siege, Pritwinarayan, the king of Gurkha, ordered that all principal persons of the town were to be put to death and that the other residents were to have their lips and noses cut off, even infants if they were not actually in their mother's arms. The lips and noses were then to be kept, as a means of counting the number of souls. Bizarrely, those who could play wind instruments were exempted. Pritwinarayan also ordered that the name of the town be changed to Nascatapoor, or Nose-cut Town. The effects were terrible.

> Many of them put an end to their lives in despair; others came in great bodies to us, in search of medicines; and it was most shocking to see so many living people with their teeth and noses resembling the skulls of the dead.

In the beginning plastic surgery developed as a way to assuage the suffering experienced by people whose faces had been disfigured through vengeance or punishment. This has given rhinokopia a particularly important place in the history of plastic surgery, as victims desperately tried to return their looks—and lives—to normal. We can see just how important facial normality is when we consider that the earliest victims weren't surrounded by mirrors, photographs and an all-pervasive media. In addition, these patients were prepared to endure surgery without pain relief and to risk dying from post-operative infection in an attempt to achieve this. It's clear from their actions that these people weren't acting out of vanity, as they would rarely have seen their own faces, but from an overwhelming desire simply to look normal and to live in their society with the 'civil inattention' that is so important to all of us.

Until the beginning of the twentieth century most facial surgery took place on the nose. In addition to mutilation by rhinokopia, the nose's prominence naturally makes it subject to damage in a wide variety of situations, including duels, accidents and warfare. The nose is also susceptible to certain 'visible' illnesses. Syphilis affects not just the genitalia but the entire body, including the face, on which it leaves a telltale disfigurement, the syphilitic nose. Before the introduction of antibiotics (following World War II) it was possible for a simple infection to eat away the tissue of the nose; early books on plastic surgery contain hundreds of photographs that show how common and severe this was. The nose can also carry visible evidence of some private habits: cocaine addicts are prone to suffering a collapse of the bridge.

The surgery performed on the nose in these early years of plastic surgery is most accurately called reconstructive plastic surgery, although those words were not used until much later. The purpose of reconstructive surgery is to return a facial feature to normal appearance, usually for visual reasons rather than to save a life. Correction of a nose mutilated by rhinokopia is a perfect example of reconstructive plastic surgery: the person could continue to live with their mutilated nose, but the psychological effects would be terrible. What they sought was a return to facial normality to allow them to live in society again and have a semblance of a normal life. We'll see the same situation occurring with the terrible facial injuries suffered by soldiers in World War I. Reconstructive surgery was the foundation of plastic surgery and continued to be its primary purpose until the cusp of the twentieth century, when surgeons began to turn their skills to help people attain *facial improvement beyond the normal*, that is, to improve a person's aesthetic appearance even though they were not actually disfigured by accident, injury or illness. But even then, the patient's psychological motivation for surgery remained the same: an overly large nose or exaggerated facial feature has the capacity, as we've seen, to destroy confidence and alter lives.

It was only at this stage that aesthetic plastic surgery really began, but it is impossible to understand aesthetic plastic surgery without looking into its origins. The thread that joins the past to the present is as much about our developing understanding of the face and its importance to human life as it is about surgical techniques.

Sushruta

The first detailed record that we have of an aesthetic plastic surgery procedure was written in about 600 BCE and describes a rhinoplasty (an operation on the nose) to correct rhinokopia. It is found in the *Sushruta Samhitá*, a surgical treatise by Sushruta, a surgeon, physician and teacher who today is revered throughout India. The following extract tells how Sushruta replaced the tip of a severed nose:

> First a leaf of a creeper, long and broad enough to fully cover the whole of the severed or clipped off part, should be gathered; and a patch of living flesh, equal in dimension to the preceding leaf, should be sliced off (from down upward) from the region of the cheek and, after scarifying it with a knife, swiftly adhered to the severed nose. Then the cool-headed physician should steadily tie it up with a bandage decent to look at and perfectly suited to the end for which it has been employed.

It might sound a bit primitive to use a leaf, but the procedure he used isn't primitive at all. Known as the skin flap, it has brought improved appearance and renewed life to people suffering from all types of wounds, mutilations and aesthetic disfigurements, and it continues to do so in certain situations. It works on the simple principle of taking a healthy flap of tissue, covered by skin, from another part of the body to cover the defect. Although the principle is simple, it's difficult to make work. The flap must retain its blood supply from the original location until new blood vessels have grown into it from the new location, otherwise the flap will die. Despite this, the skin flap remained as the mainstay of plastic surgery right up to the late twentieth century with the advent of microsurgery, which provides an immediate blood supply to the flap by directly connecting the small vessels in the flap to donor vessels near the defect.

In the procedure described above, Sushruta took a flap of skin from his patient's cheek (using the leaf as a pattern, placed on the cheek to show the size and shape required) and attached it to the nose. However, critically, part of the flap initially remained connected to the cheek. From that connection, the flap would be fed with blood until, over the course of two or three weeks, it developed its own blood supply in its new position over the nose. Only then could the connection to the cheek be severed and the flap finally stitched into place. This would have taken several operations and quite some time to perfect. In Sushruta's era, and even until quite recently in India, the procedure was performed by members of the potter caste, such as tile- or brick-makers—using adjacent skin from the face, either from the forehead or the cheek. It is referred to as the Indian method, to distinguish it from later methods that took the skin flap from more remote sites, such as the arm.

The next 2600 years of plastic surgery—and this book—are in effect the story of the development of the humble skin flap. After Sushruta, the skin flap next comes to prominence with possibly the most famous name in the history of plastic surgery, Gaspare Tagliacozzi (1545–1599). After that the skin flap descends into a colourful period lasting two centuries, characterised by intrigue, suspicion, bizarre rumours and strange happenings. It even becomes the butt of jokes and humorous writings. But just as it seems to reach its lowest point in general esteem, it is rescued from its strange past and returned to its rightful place, becoming the foundation of plastic surgery during the twentieth century. It's hard to think of other surgical procedures that had such a journey and aroused such commentary. It demonstrates the emotions that are stirred up when the human face is tampered with.

9

Adventures in anatomy

*Our life is made by the death of others. In dead
matter insensible life remains, which, reunited to
the stomachs of living beings, resumes life, both
sensual and intellectual.*

Leonardo da Vinci

All surgical procedures on humans depend upon surgeons' knowledge of human anatomy, which in turn depends upon access to and dissection of human cadavers. Human dissections have, understandably, at times been resisted and even banned in certain countries.

Bolognese bodies

In Bologna, Italy, the teaching of human anatomy using human cadaver dissection began in the fourteenth century. Dissection had also been performed there in the previous century, but the purpose had been to establish a cause of death, essentially a post-mortem. The University of Bologna regulated the activity from 1405, when a statute was passed to ensure that a maximum of one female and two male bodies were provided per medical student, paid for by the anatomist himself. Anatomy lessons had to be publicised as a way of ensuring that the numbers were met but not exceeded. As a result, over the next hundred and fifty years the anatomies changed from being teaching events for twenty or thirty students plus other scholars and interested senior members of the population to noisy and often riotous public events.

In 1442, the *podestà*, or senior official of the city, was put in charge of finding two bodies per year, each of which had to come from at least fifty kilometres outside Bologna and be from the lower class. The favoured corpses were those of criminals who had been hanged, as the body was likely to be young or middle-aged, and healthy. The law was changed again in 1561 to allow bodies from Bologna to be used, so long as they were not considered honest citizens. This change to the supply of bodies effectively gave extra political authority over the anatomies, and this increased again in 1570 when anatomy was separated from surgery and given its own chair, under political control rather than that of the scholars.

Today, anatomical dissection is performed out of sight and in hidden-away places, and its earlier appeal to the public, scholars and social elites, even sovereigns, seems strange. But performing these events was considered part of the proper function of university teaching and to witness one offered a rare and privileged glimpse into the previously hidden workings of humankind and nature. For the anatomist, selecting a part of the body that might interest selected viewers—for instance, a skull for someone interested in the workings of the mind—helped to promote both the importance of anatomy and that of the anatomist himself.

The sessions took place at the coldest time of the year, for obvious reasons, and could accommodate two hundred people, seated in four rows around the table, although it is possible that temporary structures were erected to allow more spectators. It was eventually decreed, in 1602, that there was to be only one public anatomy course per year, held during the holiday carnival period in January. Demand for corpses during this period was high, as private anatomists could also perform public sessions, provided the anatomy professor had finished and it was still carnival time. One of these public events was described as taking place in a theatre adorned with cushions and damask at the expense of the anatomist, who also provided gifts to the prior of the Doctors of Medicine, including candles from Venice, sugar cakes and 'fine gloves' on a plate of 'fine majolica'.

A potential problem for students and teachers of anatomy was disease arising from contact with the cadavers. It was obviously undesirable to lose a learned professor, so teaching dissections were frequently carried out by underlings, while the professor sat high up on a podium holding a long stick, reaching down to point out the anatomy from an elevated distance.

Bologna's anatomy theatre

The Archiginnasio palace in Bologna houses the city's anatomy theatre, the oldest in Europe after Padua's. It was probably being used by 1639. It is a place of grandeur and beauty, with high ceilings and walls of carved wood around which stand fourteen life-sized wooden statues of famous professors of anatomy. The theatre was instrumental in the birth of modern European surgery.

Today, the entrance hall to the anatomy department of the medical school in Bologna is lined on both sides with floor-to-ceiling glass cabinets filled with more than eight hundred skulls, out of a total collection of over 2000. On each is written the name of the skull's owner, the year they died, the cause of death and the region they came from. The skulls were often taken from the bodies of 'infidels' and insane people and were kept for scientific study. Many are grotesquely deformed, eroded away through to the nose as a result of infection arising from poor dental hygiene.

In the floor above the anatomy theatre is an amazing room filled with gleaming wax models of human anatomy: full bodies in perfect detail, along with half-faces, hands, legs, stomachs, and bizarre variations such as double-headed monsters. Their colours are startling, lifelike and fresh. They are simply beautiful. These were the teaching instruments of their day, made by master craftspeople, their production sometimes involving whole families who must have ended up knowing human anatomy better than the surgeons themselves. Anna Manzolini was one of the creators; she took over the family's wax-modelling workshop after her husband's death and was eventually awarded the chair of anatomical modelling from the University of Bologna in 1760.

The models were used from the mid eighteenth century to teach anatomy, and their benefits are obvious. They were readily available, unlike human bodies, and they overcame the limitations of cadaver material, which was prone to decay and could not be overly handled. Earlier attempts at three-dimensional modelling in wood and ivory gave way to wax, as it could be modelled and coloured with the extreme precision required, making it the perfect teaching material. At the height of their popularity, wax collections were prized not just as anatomical teaching aids but also for their contribution to the cultural status of a city, evidence of their owners' participation in the larger questions about human life, the working of nature and humans' understanding of the world. The use of the models in teaching declined in the late nineteenth century as anatomy aligned itself more with science than with art, and as methods of preserving cadavers, such as the use of formaldehyde and refrigeration, improved.

Galen and Vesalius

From ancient Roman times until around the middle of the sixteenth century, anatomical discoveries had been held in check by the writings of one man, Galen of Pergamum (c. 130–c. 200 CE). A massive intellect who wrote prodigiously about the human body, Galen laid out his understanding of human anatomy with some precision, even though his dissecting work was performed predominantly on Barbary macaques (commonly known as Barbary apes) due to a Roman prohibition on human dissection. But so dominant was belief in Galen's work in the following centuries that when subsequent anatomists did dissect the human body, if what they observed contradicted Galen they would either not see what was in front of them, or believe that what they were seeing was wrong. Some even suggested that any differences were due to changes in the human body since Galen's time. To propose anything new or something that differed from Galen's observations was to oppose someone with godlike status in his field, and few had the nerve to do that. Those who tried were frequently ridiculed.

Sixteenth-century Italy (Padua and Bologna in particular), however, was a place of exploration and discovery, of scientific and artistic awakening from a past filled with superstition and tradition. In this period, which unfortunately turned out to be but a brief window in time, scholarship flowed freely between art and science. Today, we see art, philosophy and anatomy as separate fields of knowledge and expertise, but in the sixteenth century they were interrelated. Anatomists used art theories such as perspective to enhance their understanding and teaching of the human body; and artists such as Leonardo da Vinci (1452–1519) and Michelangelo (1475–1564) used anatomy to ensure the accuracy of their illustrations. The great physicians of the time were deeply influenced by this interlinked society and tended to be themselves significant art collectors.

The Flemish anatomist Andreas Vesalius (1514–1564) is the person most famously associated with a challenge to Galen's authority. In 1537, at twenty-three years of age, Vesalius became professor of surgery and anatomy in Padua, and in 1539 he received access to the bodies of criminals for the purpose of dissection. As a result of his observations, Vesalius realised for the first time that Galen's work had been entirely based on the dissection of Barbary apes and other animals rather than on humans and that he had inferred human anatomy from these dissections. It was a startling discovery, but not enough to protect Vesalius from attack by those who vilified his presumption in challenging Galen. In 1540, Vesalius was invited to perform a dissection in Bologna, an event for which three corpses and six live dogs were procured. He was pitted against another anatomist, Matteo Corti, who was a believer in Galen, and he used the dissection as a forum to display his new ideas.

In 1543, Vesalius published *De humani corporis fabrica* ('On the structure of the human body'), seven volumes of clear descriptions and intricate illustrations. Rather than accepting that anatomical knowledge was best imparted by scholastic discussions of Galen's work, Vesalius instead proposed that the only way to learn anatomy was by dissection of the human body and the use of careful observation and illustration. Eventually this broke Galen's iron grip on the subject, which had stifled enquiry and progress, and became the template for anatomy teaching.

Vesalius's most famous observations were, firstly, that the human's lower jaw comprises one bone—not two separate bones, as Galen had proposed—and, secondly, that the human sternum consists of only three parts—not the seven Galen had claimed. He made many other observations, but his real legacy was his belief that careful observation and a questioning mind are integral to the study of the human body. It was the start of modern anatomy.

10

The Italian method

*We restore, repair and make whole those parts
of the face which nature has not given or which
fortune has taken away. Not so much that they
may delight the eye, but that we should buoy up
the spirit and help the mind of the afflicted.*

Gaspare Tagliacozzi

The evolution of plastic surgery from Sushruta to the present is not an unbroken line of progression; in fact, its development has been aptly described by surgeon Frank McDowell in his history of plastic surgery as a series of 'isolated peaks of accomplishment by a few individuals, connected by slender threads'.

One of these isolated 'peaks of accomplishment' occurred in Italy in the late fifteenth century, when surgeons started to experiment with the use of the skin flap for nasal reconstruction.

Gaspare Tagliacozzi

In Bologna in the mid sixteenth century, the use of the skin flap became synonymous with one of the most famous names in the history of plastic surgery, Gaspare Tagliacozzi (1545–1599).

Without doubt, Tagliacozzi is the founding father of plastic surgery, even though he lived well before it was known by that name. He was professor of anatomy and surgery at the University of Bologna, where he developed a new skin flap technique for the nose and, significantly, wrote about it, in the first textbook of plastic surgery, *De curtorum chirurgia per insitionem* ('The surgery of defects by implantations'), in 1597. This detailed, illustrated work is akin to some of today's surgical atlases, and even to this day plastic surgeons make 'pilgrimages' to Bologna to stand in front of Tagliacozzi's statue in the city's anatomy theatre, where he is posed holding a nose in his hand.

In his book, Tagliacozzi outlined step by step the exact procedure for 'restoration of deformed noses, ears and lips by skin grafting; and of the instruments and bandages used in this surgical engrafting'. It is a classic text of early surgery and created so much interest that three editions appeared in its first year of publication—as well as multiple unauthorised copies. Tagliacozzi also wrote about the relationship between facial appearance and the soul (which later gained popularity as the previously mentioned physiognomy), and he discussed aesthetic considerations in facial surgery, such as the importance of the nose in one's overall appearance and of the lips as an aesthetic and erotic feature of the face. In fact, he wrote the most well-known *raison d'être* of facial plastic surgery, which forms the epigraph to this chapter.

His words are remarkably insightful and remain unsurpassed as a summary of the guiding principles of the surgery;

they are as true today as when they were written. The desire to be relieved of psychological affliction born of facial disfigurement or disappointment remains the prime motivation for most patients of aesthetic plastic surgeons, whose role is *to relieve psychological distress through surgery*. This is what makes the discipline quite distinct among surgical specialties.

In Tagliacozzi's day, the loss of the tip of the nose was not uncommon among young men, due to the prevalence of violence, warfare and duels. Young men starting out in life are no less aware of their looks than any other group in society, and they suffer psychologically from disfigurement just like anyone else. Julius Caesar acknowledged as much when, according to Plutarch, he instructed his men to aim for the faces of the opposing cavalrymen in the Battle of Pharsalus, in 48 BCE.

The usual solution for a lost nose was a prosthetic nose tip, which could be made from various metals or papier-mâché, and was affixed to the face each morning with glue, or with laces tied around the back of the head. The sixteenth-century astronomer Tycho Brahe is known to have worn such a nose, having lost his own in a duel in 1566. He attached the prosthesis using a paste or glue; laces reputedly chafed. Of course, the nose had to be removed prior to a sneeze. It's easy to imagine the suffering that ensued from a lifetime spent wearing such a clumsy facial prosthesis, a source not only of discomfort but also of embarrassment and humiliation.

The famous surgeon Ambroise Paré, a contemporary of Tagliacozzi, described how

> a gentleman named the Cadet of Saint Thoan, who, having lost his nose and having long worn one of silver, became angry at the remark that

there was never a lack of laughing matter when he was present.

The cadet's distress led him to seek out a surgeon to restore his nose—it is unknown if this was Tagliacozzi—but, although the result was reported to be successful, Paré remained unconvinced that it was worth the pain and discomfort. We can presume patients felt differently; for example, Camillo Porzio, who during the sixteenth century received a 'new nose' from surgeons in Calabria, wrote that although he had suffered the greatest trials the operation was

> of such excellence and so marvellous that it is a great
> shame of the present century that it is not published
> and learned by all surgeons for the benefit of all.

Tagliacozzi is believed to have been conversant with the work of Sushruta and was certainly aware of local attempts at rhinoplasty by the surgeons in Calabria and by his own professor. Like Sushruta, Tagliacozzi performed rhinoplasty using a skin flap, but, whereas Sushruta had taken the skin from the cheek and later practitioners had taken it from the forehead, Tagliacozzi chose not to use skin adjacent to the nose, but rather skin from the inner side of the upper arm. He was not the first surgeon to do this, but his careful recording and illustration of the technique in his book, and his belief in the procedure, has meant that his name is the one associated with this method, which became known as the Italian method.

Although the arms seem a long way from the nose, there are significant advantages in using them: the upper arm is large enough to provide sufficient skin; and its skin is soft and not too hairy, can be obtained without too much danger or discomfort to the patient, and is capable of being separated from the underlying tissue without difficulty. (Tagliacozzi didn't think the forehead skin well suited, as it has a muscle situated immediately beneath.) Significantly, using the upper arm meant no scar was left on the forehead or cheek, ensuring that the surgery was concealed and the patient free from any stigma relating either to the original deformity or to the surgery itself. In this Tagliacozzi demonstrated once again his understanding of the psychological dimension of his work.

Transferring skin from the upper arm to the nose was more complicated than just swinging it across from the cheek or forehead, however. What it meant was that the arm had to be fixed to the face and scalp for the 'contact stage' of the flap transfer—that is, until the flap had developed its own secure blood supply at the site of implantation on the face—a period of between fourteen and twenty days. To achieve this, Tagliacozzi devised a complicated leather harness support system that held the patient's inner arm firmly pressed against the nose, with the wrist and hand resting on top of the head. His engravings of patients held in this pose are some of the most famous illustrations in the history of surgery and give a clear indication of what an uncomfortable process this must have been.

In fact, all six steps of the surgery would have been distressingly painful. There was a minimum interval of fourteen days between most steps. The skin flap would be dissected from the upper arm (lifted from the underlying tissue and a piece of linen cloth placed under it to ensure separation) but left attached at both ends. Then the upper end of the flap would be severed to allow the blood supply from the lower end to strengthen so that the flap could be trained—that is, given time to gain strength and for the inner surface to harden. The upper end of

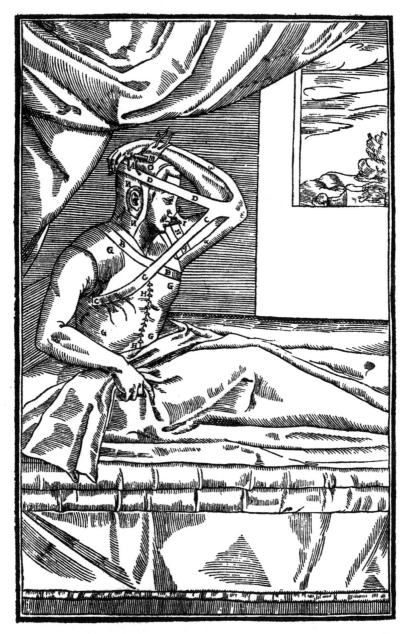

Illustration from Tagliacozzi's book De curtorum chirurgia, *showing his famous harness devised to keep stable contact between the upper arm and the nose for the period of implantation, up to twenty-one days.*

the flap would then be fixed in its new position on the nose, and, after it had gained a new blood supply from the nose, it was finally severed from its attachment to the arm. Rosewater and eggwhite were used to reduce inflammation. The final steps involved shaping the skin flap to fit the nose and stitching it in place. For the next two years the patient would wear nasal tubes and moulds to ensure clear airways and correct shaping. He would end up with a nose that was lighter in colour and softer than the original, but in time it would harden and look more natural.

In total, the operation took between ninety-one and a hundred and thirty-six days, depending on the age of the patient and the season. Tagliacozzi wrote that spring was the best season for healing, winter the worst. The complete lack of anaesthesia or antisepsis, and the patient's discomfort in the harness, clearly display the strength of the desire for facial normality that motivated these patients.

As we have seen, Bologna in the sixteenth century, full of scientific and artistic endeavour, was the perfect environment for exploratory thinking—and for plastic surgery. However, at the same time, rhinoplasty was a source of controversy among surgeons: even the greatest dismissed, criticised or misunderstood it. It was seen as a form of grafting—a practice associated with plants, not human beings—and provoked out-rage. Allegations and rumours of supernatural dabblings were levelled at Tagliacozzi that continued for the rest his life, and for centuries after his death. Science may briefly have been in the ascendant, but the popular mind was still a ferment of belief in mystical forces, the devil, amulets, astrology and portents. Tagliacozzi's misfortune was to have had an idea centuries before its time.

Burying Tagliacozzi

At Tagliacozzi's funeral in 1599, humanist and poet Muzio Piacentini gave the oration, using what later proved to be fateful words:

> Against reluctant nature's will, he made these mutilated features whole again in such a fashion that they were once more natural ornaments of the face, as they had been before; so that even though people looked with lynx eyes, they could see no scars; there was apparent no trace, not even the slightest, of the parts of the human visage having been lost.

Tagliacozzi was buried in the Church of San Giovanni Battista, but not long afterwards his body was dug up and reinterred outside the church walls. The reason given at the time was that the nuns of the church had heard a voice during the night telling them that Tagliacozzi had been damned. A tribunal of the Inquisition was called, which returned Tagliacozzi's body to its original grave, exonerated him and did what it could to restore his name and good reputation.

This story, re-told through the ages, was used to demonstrate the Church's opposition to surgery, and Tagliacozzi's 'face-changing' surgery in particular.

However, recent historical research has shed new light on the episode, suggesting that Tagliacozzi's enemies, rather than the Catholic Church, may have been responsible. His enemies had been making accusations of impiety and magic against him because they were outraged by his skin grafting and resented his success in an activity that they considered unnatural. That the grafting changed the patient's face, given by God, had made matters worse. It is possible that the funeral oration that had praised Tagliacozzi's work so highly had actually reignited these concerns and inspired the exhumation.

Strange stories

Despite his careful work, rhinoplasty failed to flourish after Tagliacozzi's death, largely due to a change in the intellectual climate in Italy and a decline in the overall popularity of surgery. Anatomy and human dissection at times descended into grotesque spectacle, even being transformed into social events attended by huge, well-dressed audiences and culminating in lavish balls stretching into the night. Tagliacozzi's technique fell victim to lurid rumours and became embroiled in competition with other surgical theories through the following centuries. Indeed, the surgeon Joseph Constantine Carpue (1764–1846), writing in 1816, claimed that by the time of Tagliacozzi's theories' eventual resurrection, which occurred during the nineteenth century, his work was mentioned 'only as an historical curiosity or a joking tale'.

The rumours included tales of bad results from Tagliacozzi's rhinoplasty: ice-cold or red nose tips, some that putrefied and died, and others that were so fragile that they couldn't be touched or blown for fear of dropping right off. Some surgeons wrote that the procedure was difficult, that it used muscle or flesh as well as skin, and that the graft took forty days to become properly attached. As inaccurate information took these surgeons further away from Tagliacozzi's original technique, they reported the results to be ineffective and not worth the effort. With Tagliacozzi dead and his book scarce, the inaccuracies weren't corrected.

'Sympathetic nose', or 'sympathetic slave', stories were among the strangest to circulate. There was a persistent idea that instead of using their own skin, patients could use the skin of another person to repair their nose. These days, of course, we know this is impossible, as the body naturally rejects foreign material—skin grafts using skin from another person will die after a week or two—but at the time the immune system wasn't understood. Slaves were said to be especially useful as 'donors', although they presumably would have had little choice in the matter. The problem was, according to the stories, that when the slave died so did their donated skin, wherever in the world it happened to be. Upon the slave's death, the recipient would suddenly find themselves with a decaying nose. This, it was alleged, was due to a sympathetic connection that endured between the donor and their distant skin, preventing the skin from ever becoming a true part of the recipient. Despite the obvious difficulties of attaching another person's arm to your nose, immobilised, for the period required—a point specifically made by Tagliacozzi, who had considered the technique when use of another's skin was suggested—these strange stories developed a life of their own, as different writers embellished them with eyewitness accounts of putrefying noses.

The stories were able to become so widespread because of the popularity of theories of sympathetic surgery, which flourished especially around the early seventeenth century. 'Sympathetic doctors' believed that the body was infused with a magnetic spirit, or *mumia*, which extended to every part. If you took the skin off one body and grafted it onto another, the spiritual bond would remain with the original donor, and the skin would die when that original donor died. The theory was vigorously opposed by other doctors, who saw it as the work of the devil. In an escalating battle to protect the validity of their theory and to prove that they weren't practising the devil's work, sympathetic doctors eagerly promoted stories of nose death occurring after the donor's death. In fact, the stranger the story, the more it proved their case, so they didn't hold back.

The whole dispute, and the vehemence on each side, is hard for us to understand today, but it was part of the battle for acceptance of surgery in general and between competing theories in particular. Unfortunately for Tagliacozzi, his name was so connected to the idea of rhinoplasty that any nose story, no matter how fanciful, implicated him in some way. As time went on, the tales spread and became part of popular culture, making nose surgery a perfect target for humorists, who lampooned it mercilessly. British writers such as William Congreve, Samuel Butler and the founders of *The Spectator* magazine, Joseph Addison and Richard Steele, incorporated the idea of skin flaps and Tagliacozzi (whom they called Taliacotius) into their writing, bawdily sending up the Italian's ideas. For example, an article in *The Tatler* in December 1710 told the following tale:

> The Sympathy betwixt the Nose and its Parent was very extraordinary. *Hudibrass* has told us, that when the Porter [donor] died the Nose dropped of Course, in which Case it was always usual to return the Nose, in order to have it interred with its first Owner. The Nose was likewise affected by the Pain as well as Death of the Original Proprietor. An eminent Instance of this Nature happened to three *Spaniards*, whose Noses were all made out of the same Piece of Brawn. They found them one Day shoot and swell extremely; upon which they sent to know how the Porter did, and heard upon Enquiry, that the Parent of the Noses had been severely kicked

the Day before, and that the Porter kept is [*sic*] Bed on Account of the Bruises it had received …

On the other Hand, if any Thing went amiss with the Nose, the Porter felt the Effects of it, insomuch that it was generally articled with the Patient, that he should … on no Pretence what soever smell Pepper, or eat Mustard; on which Occasion the Part where the Incision had been made was seized with unspeakable Twinges and Prickings.

Another example is found in the first part of Samuel Butler's poem *Hudibras* (mentioned in the story above) and was used as a warning to young men that they should not live recklessly, as there was 'a Taliacotius at the corner of every street'. It shows just how familiar Tagliacozzi's name was a century after his death, and how entangled his reputation had become with ludicrous stories and humour over that time.

> So learned Taliacotius from
> The brawny part of the porter's bum,
> Cut supplemental noses, which
> Wou'd last as long as parent breech;
> But when the date of Nock was out,
> Off drop'd the sympathetic snout.

A century after Butler's poem, Tagliacozzi's method suddenly received renewed credibility. It came about through another strange—but this time true—story. In October 1794 a letter from 'B L' appeared in the *Gentleman's Magazine* in London, relating the tale of Cowasjee, a bullock driver with the British army whose nose and hand had been cut off when he was taken prisoner by a sultan in India. A 'very curious' operation was performed on Cowasjee following his release, namely affixing a new nose to his face using a skin flap from his forehead. B L reported:

> This operation is very generally successful. The artificial nose is secure, and looks nearly as well as the natural one; nor is the scar on the forehead very observable after a length of time.

Of course, it was still lampooned and a later account, from 1798, described Cowasjee's nose more colourfully and included a reference to Butler's parodying words about Tagliacozzi.

> The sufferer applied to the great restorer of *Hindoostan* noses, and a new one, equal to all the uses of its predecessor, immediately rose in its place. It can sneeze smartly, distinguish good from bad smells, bear the most provoking lug, or being well blown without danger of falling into the handkerchief. It will last the life of the wearer; nor like the *Taliacotian*, need he fear,
>
>> That when the date of *Nock* is out,
>> The drop of sympathetic snout.

Rhinoplasty's revival

The appearance of the story of Cowasjee, the humble bullock driver, was an important turning point for plastic surgery, and for rhinoplasty in Europe. It caught the attention of British surgeon Joseph Constantine Carpue, a well-connected friend of the king and of Sir Joseph Banks, president of the Royal Society. Carpue wrote to various contacts in India and learnt that these operations were commonly performed and had been since time immemorial. They were indeed usually successful and were practised (as they had been in Sushruta's day) by the caste of potters.

Carpue began a long process of learning and experimentation, using both the Indian method (with forehead skin) and the Italian method (with skin from the upper arm). He then performed two well-documented operations on British army officers, in 1814 and 1815, using the Indian technique. One of the men had lost his nose to mercury treatment for a liver disease, the other to a sword. Carpue's record of the operations, *An Account of Two Successful Operations for Restoring a Lost Nose from the Integuments of the Forehead*, was published in London in 1816, complete with illustrations by one of the best engravers of the day, Charles Turner. It made, according to the surgeon subsequently responsible for its translation into German, 'an instant and profound impression throughout Britain and the Continent'. Not only did it lead to a revival of interest in rhinoplasty across Europe, but it also restored Tagliacozzi's reputation, as Carpue showed in detail how unjustly Tagliacozzi had been treated over the past two centuries, decrying the way in which his reputation had been denigrated to such an extent that his work had become 'classed with the exploits of Jack the Giant-killer and spoken of only to amuse children'.

However, even being a famous surgeon whose work was encouraged by an interested prince regent, later George IV, didn't allow Carpue to escape the lampoonists' wit. A marble bust of him, completed in 1847, sits on a plinth inscribed with words from the poem 'Mary's Ghost: A pathetic ballad' (1827), by the humorist Thomas Hood, in which a disembodied ghost complains that her body has been taken by body snatchers:

I can't tell where my head is gone.
But Dr Carpue can;
As for my trunk, it's all packed up
To go by Pickford's van.

While Carpue was using the Indian method, German surgeon Karl Ferdinand von Graefe was practising Tagliacozzi's Italian method. In his foreword to the German edition of Carpue's *Account*, which he arranged himself, Graefe described his own work as

> a completely successful attempt, not only to rescue the Italian method from oblivion, but also to transplant it from Italy, which it had never left, onto German soil, where, according to the testimony of all the writers, it had never been tried.

Graefe's edition of Carpue's book added to the rebirth of European restorative nose surgery. In the foreword he praised Tagliacozzi's method for its avoidance of a disfiguring forehead scar and its 'firmer growth and more definitive shape', continuing:

> I will at present only mention that the part taken from the arm of my good patient has grown firmly to the face, that it grew vigorously, has warmth and feeling, that the scar closed well, that the colour is now entirely harmonious with the face; that further, the nostrils are of natural size and shape, that the septum, and the overall shape of the nose are very satisfying, and that the new nose will be able to perform all the functions of its predecessor.

A few years later, in 1818, Graefe wrote his own book on rhino-plasty, entitled *Rhinoplastik*. Many believe this is the first use of the word 'plastic' in conjunction with this type of surgery.

The persistent black humour—and ghoulish writings—provoked by facial surgery and the use of the skin flap are testimony to the unease they created. The unease persists today: even though surgery has become a common part of our lives during the twentieth and twenty-first centuries, some discomfort is still expressed when a face is altered or actually re-created—as in contemporary face transplants. Some people raise the same objections that were voiced against early heart transplants in the late 1960s: that the surgery interferes with a person's identity and soul.

During the nineteenth century Tagaliacozzi's work was finally restored to its rightful position of respect. His technique was widely used during the twentieth century by revered pioneers in plastic surgery. Today, his portrait appears in the logo of the American Board of Plastic Surgery and his famous illustration of a patient in a harness during the restoration of his nose forms part of the emblem of the American Association of Plastic Surgeons.

11

World War I

*When you change a man's face, you almost change
a man's person, his behaviour, and sometimes even
his basic talents and abilities.*

Maxwell Maltz

World War I was a major event in the development of facial surgery. It's worth remembering that at the time of the war, plastic surgery as a speciality did not exist—a situation changed by that conflict. The surgeon's work raised the interesting question: at what point does reconstructive surgery become aesthetic? We would now describe this as being different points along a continuum, but during the war surgeons who initially did not believe they worked in the realm of aesthetic considerations began to understand how inextricably their surgery affected their patients' subsequent fate. Some went further and realised that their work was an art as well as a science. Even though they were not performing aesthetic surgery in the sense that we now know it, of enhancing appearance, they were increasingly aware of the importance of aesthetics in what they did.

Because of the new weaponry that came into use during the war, particularly shrapnel and machine guns, surgeons were suddenly confronted with injuries on a scale and intensity never seen before. Soldiers didn't understand the damage that the new weapons could cause, especially to the face; Fred Albee, a US surgeon who operated on the wounded in France, wrote that they

> failed to understand the menace of the machine gun. They seemed to think they could pop their heads up over a trench and move quickly enough to dodge the hail of machine-gun bullets.

The massive, unprecedented types of injuries they received forced surgeons to improvise, experiment and develop new techniques. Contemporary photographs and illustrations show soldiers with entire parts of their faces missing; sometimes even half the face could be completely blown away without death resulting immediately.

Facial wounds became known as being the most traumatic of war injuries. This was because they affected the entire identity and future life of the victim. Some men committed suicide because of their destroyed face, while others suffered so deep an anguish at the prospect of living with such disfigurements that they chose instead to hide away, out of the sight of other people. Stories abound of children filled with fear at the sight of their father, and of relationships destroyed. One officer was said to have made the humane decision to shoot a severely facially wounded soldier, knowing that effectively his 'life' had ended at the moment of impact.

Of course, the surgery that the soldiers received was reconstructive rather than aesthetic, but surgeons quickly noticed that restoring a face to mere functionality was not enough; for the men's happiness and fulfilment in their future life it also had to be as close to normal as possible. These young men, not even in their prime, had to go back to their parents, partners and children after the war, returning to normal life, working and supporting their families. If they aroused pity or horror (as many did), a descent into depression and increasing isolation quickly followed.

Face fixing

Varaztad Kazanjian, a US dentist volunteer during the war, became famous in plastic surgery history for rebuilding the face of Lance Corporal Fred Snowdon, who had lost his mouth, chin and jaw to a shell. Kazanjian, who worked on more than three thousand such cases, recognised the necessity of restoration of function, but also of aesthetic normality. He observed that 'it was the great need of the time that evolved the techniques that made it possible for injured men to speak again, to look something like they had before'.

The 'stream of wounded men' and their terrible facial injuries were, at first, embarrassing to general surgeons as they struggled to help those with 'half their faces literally blown to pieces, with the skin left hanging in shreds and the jawbones crushed to a pulp that felt like sand under your fingers'. They stitched up the gaping wounds, but closing the gap without replacing the lost tissue meant the face was not rebuilt aesthetically. From this desperate need, Sushruta's and Tagliacozzi's humble skin flap was developed further.

New Zealand–born surgeon Harold Gillies (1882–1960) was most famously associated with this development. In fact, in his book *Plastic Surgery of the Face* (1920), Gillies acknowledged the early work of the Indian surgeons and Tagliacozzi, calling the skin flap 'the ABC of the surgeon's work', which it surely was. Many of the photographs in his book, showing patients with flaps bringing skin up to their face, are highly reminiscent of Tagliacozzi's illustrations of patients 'harnessed' to hold their upper arm and nose together. During the war Gillies operated at the Cambridge Hospital in Aldershot and then at Queen's Hospital, Sidcup, which was established in August 1917 specifically to cope with the mass of facial injuries coming in from the trenches. Within a year the hospital and its nearby satellites extended to 1000 beds, all filled. Sidcup became known as the birthplace of modern plastic surgery.

The number of wounds that the doctors dealt with at the time is staggering: on one day alone, following the Battle of the Somme, Gillies was sent 2000 patients. He described his days and nights as filled with the problems of the wounded, his wards filled with bed after bed of men unable to speak, eat, taste, many unable to see and nearly all unable to sleep. Some begged to be killed, others willed themselves to die, and still others isolated themselves. Mirrors were banned: those who had been blinded seemed to keep up their spirits better than those who could see. The worst two wards were called, by the other patients, the Chamber of Horrors.

One of Gillies's patients, a handsome young corporal, talked constantly in the ward about his girlfriend. She wrote to him daily, but he told her not to visit while his face was bandaged, as he didn't want to scare her with his 'Egyptian mummy' appearance. Although mirrors were banned from the ward, he had held on to his small shaving mirror. When he finally saw what his face looked like, he collapsed.

> All hope of allowing his girl to visit him died with that forbidden glimpse. From then on he insisted on being screened from the rest of the ward patients. When at long last he went home, it was to lead the life of a recluse.

Injuries illustrated

At the outbreak of World War I, artist Henry Tonks (1862–1937) was teaching at the Slade School of Fine Arts in London. He had trained as a surgeon; in fact, he had been a surgical assistant to Frederick Treves, the surgeon who helped Joseph Merrick (perhaps better known as the 'Elephant Man'), and he had illustrated one of Treves's articles about the dissection of two rhinoceroses from London Zoo. During the war, Tonks assisted Harold Gillies in developing the idea of the nexus between art and surgery. He observed Gillies's work, using his artistic talents to depict the deformities encountered and techniques applied. His pastel drawings of the servicemen that Gillies operated on are some of the most famous illustrations of the war, leaving no-one in any doubt of the horrors suffered by the soldiers and the enormous task faced by Gillies and his colleagues each day.

Gillies calmed the wounded men, joking with them and assuring them that they'd have 'as good a face as most of us before we're finished with you'. He knew how important it was for their recovery that they could hope to look as normal as possible. Gillies thought about this and was 'uplifted by the idea that the activities of a plastic surgeon were essentially creative, that they demanded the vision and the insight of an artist'. He named it 'a strange new art', as indeed it was.

Gillies developed a renowned technique, the tubed pedicle, which improved the use and versatility of the skin flap by strengthening its critical blood supply and reach. The idea came to Gillies while he was lifting a strip of skin off a patient's shoulder and noticed that it had a natural tendency to curl inwards rather than stay flat. Using this inclination, he stitched the curled edges of the strip together, creating a tube of living tissue that could be used as a temporary bridge, producing a blood supply between the donor site and the flap. The tubed pedicle allowed a greater distance between the donor and the recipient sites and made it easier to swing large amounts of skin up from the back or chest for use on the face. The closed tube was also stronger than a single flap of skin and, being sealed off, was less prone to infection and degeneration over time, two problems that had been encountered by skin flap surgeons. A further ingenious advance with the tubed pedicle was called 'waltzing the flap'. This allowed skin from an undamaged donor area remote from the face to be moved gradually, in multiple stages, up the body to the final site, each end being severed in turn and reattached to a point closer to the face.

The tubed pedicle was enormously important and was taken around the world by the many surgeons who worked with Gillies during the war years. It only became obsolete with the advent of microsurgery in the 1970s, which gives surgical results and convenience beyond anything Gillies could have imagined. But even that hasn't meant the end of skin flap surgery. It is still practised today following surgery for skin cancers, where small local flaps are employed, especially on the face, using a variation of the Indian method. It is also used when microsurgery isn't available, and at a very sophisticated level in the most technically advanced face lifts.

The idea that surgery and art could intersect was not immediately accepted by other surgeons, but Harold Gillies, having encountered so much facial trauma, realised the truth of Tagliacozzi's dictum that a key purpose of this surgery should be to 'buoy up the spirit and help the mind of the afflicted'. In 1957, towards the end of his life, Gillies co-authored a work with a US plastic surgeon later to be famous in his own right, D Ralph Millard Jr. He called it *The Principles and Art of Plastic Surgery*.

Ironically, during World War II an equally important surgical role was played by Gillies's younger cousin, and fellow New Zealander, Sir Archibald McIndoe. The two cousins started working together in the United Kingdom before the war, where Gillies stressed to his young relative the importance of perfect stitching to plastic surgery. He even suggested using pillowcases or old felt hats until perfection had been achieved. In 1939, the two cousins made up half the total number of plastic surgeons working full time in the United Kingdom; that is, four surgeons. When war was announced the government, having learnt the importance of plastic surgery from the previous war, set up four plastic surgery centres, one for each surgeon.

McIndoe chose the Queen Victoria Hospital in East Grinstead, where he ended up dealing with the bulk of the casualties, the worst of them in the famous Ward Three. Fondly known collectively as his 'guinea pigs', his patients were mostly young airmen who had suffered terrible burns. McIndoe became renowned for his saline bath treatments and skin grafting to treat the burns.

From the first he made sure that patients were cared for psychologically as well as physically, as he understood how difficult it was going to be for these young men to rebuild their confidence with such badly damaged faces. He ensured the nurses understood the importance of caring for the patient's mental state and he even changed the interior colour scheme from the government's cream and brown to cheerier greens and pinks with chintz curtains. Inside Ward Three he fostered an atmosphere free of unnecessary rules and without segregation by rank or status.

Famously, he also ensured that the locals in East Grinstead were prepared for the disfigured faces and bodies that would soon be appearing on their streets. He actively encouraged the townspeople to socialise with the airmen as a first step to rebuilding their social confidence. It must have been a challenge for some of the locals. An artist who visited the hospital expressed astonishment at seeing men playing football with flap and tube grafts joining their shoulder to their face.

After the war, McIndoe developed a strong aesthetic practice and contributed to lower eyelid surgery and face lift techniques, as well as to reconstructive surgery.

Tin Noses Shop

Unfortunately, despite the best efforts of surgeons like Harold Gillies, the appalling disfigurements suffered by some World War I soldiers meant that their faces could not be made aesthetically acceptable. For those men, whose lives had been saved but who remained hideous to look at, the answer was a facial mask. The sculptor Francis Derwent Wood (1871–1926) created a workshop in the Third London General Hospital called the Masks for Facial Disfigurement Department, known by the soldiers as the Tin Noses Shop. He upgraded the masks given to the men, which were initially made of rubber, to lightweight metal and painted them with oils in an attempt to recreate a facial likeness of each soldier, using prewar photographs as guides. To our eyes the masks look grotesque, but by hiding the disfigurement which was even worse they allowed the soldiers to regain their lives.

> My cases are generally extreme cases that plastic surgery has, perforce, abandoned; but as in plastic surgery, the psychological effect is the same. The patient acquires his old self-respect, self-assurance, self-reliance … takes once more to a pride in his personal appearance. His presence is no longer a source of melancholy to himself nor of sadness to his relatives and friends.

Wood's work was another attempt—albeit a slightly forlorn one—to 'buoy up the spirit and help the mind' of the facially afflicted. His observation that facial appearance matters not just to the person but also to the people around them would be confirmed later in the twentieth century by psychological studies using brain scan technology.

Facial masks developed further after 1917 when US sculptor Anna Coleman Ladd opened the Studio for Portrait Masks in Paris under the auspices of the American Red Cross. Expanding Wood's work, she also tried to assist men so that they could continue their lives and, most importantly, earn their living after the war.

Sadly, it is believed that many of the men who were forced to wear masks ended up choosing to work in darkness and solitude, with many making their living as film projectionists.

Face transplants

One can only imagine Gillies's response if he had lived long enough to witness the twenty-first century's face transplants. The first full face transplant in the world was performed in Spain in March 2010. According to *The Guardian* in July of that year, the thirty-one-year-old recipient had accidentally shot himself in the face five years earlier and before the transplant had been unable to eat or breathe properly. Shortly after the transplant he was able to drink, eat soft food and shave. His sister said that he was looking forward to

> little things, like walking down the street without anyone looking at him, or sitting down for a meal with his family. Doing things that all of us do on a normal day.

A year later, in the United States, another full face transplant was carried out successfully. *The Australian* reported in May 2011 that the recipient, twenty-six-year-old Dallas Wiens, had touched an electrical wire while in a cherry picker, painting a church, and his face had been burnt off. Following his transplant, he first noticed simple experiences such as being able to breathe properly through his nose and to smell food. He was eager to resume normal life as soon as his appearance would enable him to do so. He commented with pride on the fact that his young daughter had called him handsome.

Operation Mend

The importance of restoring more than health and function to a face has been recognised by a philanthropic program called Operation Mend at the medical centre of the University of California, Los Angeles, for US soldiers returning from the Iraq and Afghanistan conflicts. While military hospitals provide excellent care in restoring health, their focus has not extended to restoring appearance. Operation Mend offers free aesthetic surgery to service members who have suffered disfiguring facial injuries. Echoing the experience of the soldiers of World War I, a serviceman from Afghanistan who was severely burnt described having become a recluse, hiding behind hooded sweatshirts, baseball caps and dark glasses on the rare occasions he went out. According to *The New York Times* in January 2012, his surgery at Operation Mend restored 'not just a semblance of his former visage, but also a healthy chunk of his self confidence'.

The prominence given by the media to face transplants is testimony to the special way in which they affect us. Other transplants are invisible, but with faces the transplant goes to the centre of the donor's and the recipient's identities. As mentioned earlier, this idea of possibly transplanting identity along with an organ also arose with heart transplants, as the heart is another part of the body associated with emotion. There's almost a feeling of social unease around face transplants similar to that which Tagliacozzi experienced with his rhinoplasties, and this is compounded by the commonly expressed concern that the recipient will look like the donor. This, fortunately, is not the case, as the transplanted face covers the underlying structure of the recipient's bones and muscles, which ensures that a 'new' face is created.

Full face transplants belong to the realm of microsurgery and are a quantum leap from the skin flap, but World War I was itself responsible for an earlier quantum leap, forcing accelerated learning that alerted surgeons to the wider possibilities of facial surgery. Some went back to their practices after the war and started experimenting and writing, using what they'd learnt from the war to improve outcomes for their own patients. But still, it wasn't until the end of World War II that plastic surgery—including aesthetic plastic surgery—spread across society and entered a phase of unprecedented growth.

12

Surgery for the public

*A good face they say, is a letter of recommendation.
O Nature, Nature, why art thou so dishonest, as
ever to send men with these false recommendations
into the World!*

Henry Fielding

hen plastic surgery finally spread into the public
domain, it started with the procedure we've followed through the centuries, from Sushruta to
Tagliacozzi to Carpue: rhinoplasty. By the closing days of the
nineteenth century, when this occurred, the introduction of
antisepsis and the adoption of anaesthesia had made surgery
not only safer but also bearable. The birth of anaesthesia is
usually dated to an operation by the dentist William Thomas
Green Morton in October 1846, when he removed some teeth
after administering inhaled ether to his patient, a process he

repeated the following day—with more success—to remove a fatty tumour from the arm of a patient. This miracle of unconsciousness without death was a critical step that allowed patients and doctors alike to view surgery as something other than an extreme act. In 1867, antisepsis followed, when Joseph Lister developed a model of cleansing using carbolic acid before and after surgery. His 'germ theory', the notion of infection by microorganism, replaced the earlier idea that infection was spread by miasma, or bad air. Germ theory was ridiculed at first but it gradually became accepted by the medical fraternity.

Attitudes themselves had also changed and the individual in society—other than the very poor—had a newfound freedom that enabled them to make decisions about their lives and beliefs. Following the spread of Enlightenment ideas in the eighteenth century, established orthodoxies had been challenged and reason, rather than religion, moved to the centre of thinking. Old structures of authority, such as the Church and paternalistic hierarchies in society, had less influence over how people thought. It had been a long but inexorable process. The French Revolution (1789–1799) and the later wave of revolutions across Europe in the mid nineteenth century saw people fighting for ideas such as liberty, equality and fraternity, which would have been considered unthinkable in the earlier rigidly structured societies. These ideas, which had swept across the United States, England, Scotland and other European countries, arrived with the rise of a new middle-class, town-living people with money and independence. The American Declaration of Independence (1776) was just one of many writings to have spelt out the new thinking: humans were created equal, they had certain unalienable rights, and one of these was the pursuit of happiness—a life that fulfilled the individual's personal desires and expectations. So when painless, safer surgery became available to this large and liberated group, there was immediate interest in what it could provide. They had the freedom to act, a desire to live better lives, the money to pay for it, and an acceptance that problems were not just to be accepted as God-given but could be altered by their own will and actions.

Operating on the psyche

Early practitioners offering aesthetic plastic surgery to the public quickly became fascinated with the psychological dimensions of their work and, like Harold Gillies, came to realise the importance of a 'normal' face. If initially they believed that they were just performing surgery, they soon understood that they were also mending lives.

Surgeon Charles H Willi (c. 1882–1972), practising in London in the first decades of the twentieth century, was visited by a man and his twenty-year-old son, who had protruding ears. The young man had become obsessed with his ears to the point that when they were out motoring and passed another car he would ask, 'Did you see the people looking at my ears?' Eventually he had refused to leave home and his father feared that he would commit suicide. Fortunately, when his ears were fixed, the problem was resolved. We will never know whether people in other cars really did stare at his ears—it seems unlikely—but he had advanced to the stage of both expecting and dreading their stares, and that was enough to destroy his happiness.

John Orlando Roe (1848–1915), one of the most famous names in aesthetic surgery and known as the father of aesthetic rhinoplasty, was an otolaryngologist (commonly known as an ear, nose and throat surgeon) who practised in New York. His papers on aesthetic rhinoplasty are considered to form the 'start of corrective aesthetic rhinoplasty'. In 1905, he wrote:

> We are able to relieve patients of a condition which would remain a life-long mark of disfigurement, constantly observed, forming a never-ceasing source of embarrassment and mental distress to themselves, amounting, in many cases, to positive torture, as well as often causing them to be objects of greater or less aversion to others.
>
> It will be a surprise to any physician, who will take the trouble to investigate the subject, to find how many brilliant lives, how many noble personalities, and how much valuable talent have been, so to speak, buried from human eyes, lost to the world and society, by reason of the embarrassment and mortification caused by the conscious, or in some cases, the unconscious influence of some physical infirmity or deformity or unsightly blemish.

Early demand was high, from males and females of all ages. The nose was the focus for reasons that were not dissimilar to those of centuries earlier: patients had congenital deformities that left them with misshaped noses; had been kicked by a horse or fallen off one; had suffered a bicycle, automobile, cart or sporting accident, a fall or fight; had been dropped as a child; or, in one case, had been attacked by highwaymen. As usual, however, infection was a major cause of nasal disfigurement. Patients with lupus could look literally as if their nose had been bitten off by a wolf, and those with syphilis could be identified by the collapse of the bridge of their nose, the 'saddle nose'.

Roe's near contemporary Jacques Joseph (1865–1934), an equally famous name in early rhinoplasty, was a professor of orthopaedics at Berlin's renowned Charité Hospital who published and taught extensively and whose work became known in the 1920s and early 1930s. In 1904, he wrote some of the first modern medical acknowledgements of the distress suffered by such patients and their 'urgent desire to become free and unconstrained'.

Ageing and early face lifts

As these surgeons came to realise, the extent of psychological distress suffered by people with facial abnormalities doesn't necessarily correlate with the objective size of the deformity. This is a profound observation, because those who are not afflicted might expect the opposite to be the case. Another vital recognition at the time was of the material loss arising from facial distress. In an early nod to pulchronomics—the economic advantages of looking attractive—there was pressure on people in the early twentieth century to look younger in order to retain their jobs in a competitive marketplace; this was a key factor in the early popularity of rejuvenation surgery. And so, at the same time that rhinoplasty was 'going public', some surgeons began to turn their attention to the ageing process and the development of rejuvenation surgery.

Age-related changes of the face are misunderstood. The word 'wrinkles' is the first that comes to mind when most people think about facial ageing, but if you really look at the faces of older people it becomes quite obvious that most don't have masses of wrinkles, but all have undergone similar changes in their facial shape, which is due to the laxity of the facial tissues during the ageing process. The recogniseable shape of the ageing face is the reason a middle-aged person with unwrinkled skin still looks their age. It's also what creates a certain sameness as people get older. For most people, wrinkles tend to appear later, beyond middle age, as part of more advanced ageing.

Artist William Hogarth, ever observant, noticed this. He saw that ageing is mostly about the loss of pleasing lines and sweeping planes, that the face breaks up into 'dented shapes' and that increasing age lays on 'strokes and cuts'. It's a good way of putting it. He also observed that the main change occurs around the muscles, a function of their 'many repeated move-ments'. That observation put him about two hundred years ahead of the anatomists. The dents, strokes and cuts—which are now called grooves, furrows and folds—are what make us look tired and careworn with age. The skin itself also ages, mainly from environmental factors such as sun exposure, and this adds to the look of age but does not create it.

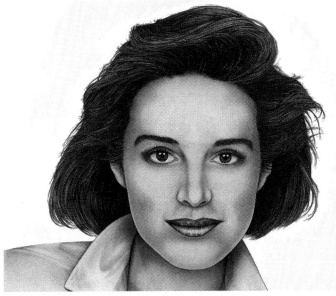

Image 1: The smooth facial contours of youth.

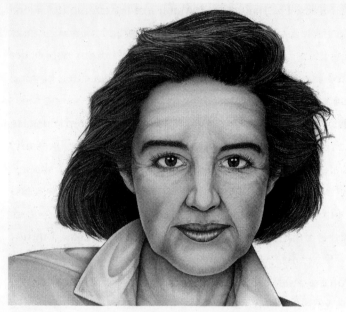

Image 2: The 'tired look' of middle age, the result of changed facial shape.

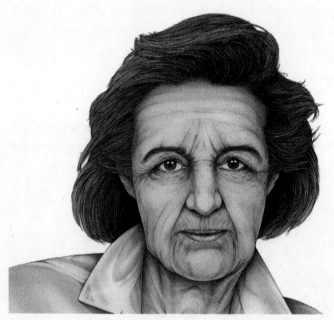

Image 3: Old age brings the appearance of wrinkles and more advanced facial laxity.

It has been more than a century since rejuvenation surgery was first attempted. It was an exciting start: the pioneer surgeons were delighted with their results and especially interested by the psychological lift their patients experienced as a result of looking younger. But in the early days the focus was on the eradication of wrinkles and sagging, and the results, although definitely showing improvement, were not necessarily natural-looking.

The first patients, of course, had no expectations whatsoever. The whole idea of rejuvenation was entirely new, so they were grateful for any benefit in their appearance. By the time rejuvenation surgery had advanced to the stage of providing subtle and natural results, in the late 1980s and 1990s, expectations were quite different. By then patients were becoming familiar with the good and bad of rejuvenation surgery. Today, most surgeons and patients share the goals of undetectable surgery and a totally natural-looking result.

The earliest text on the subject is usually attributed to a maverick surgeon from Chicago, Charles Conrad Miller, who published *The Correction of Featural Imperfections* in 1907. A colourful figure, Miller described his eyelid rejuvenation procedure as simple and able to be performed painlessly, which he qualified somewhat by adding that 'by painlessly, I do not mean that the patient is hanging on to the table with both hands and praying for the early conclusion of the ordeal'.

Suzanne Noël

One of the most fascinating early plastic surgeons to peform rejuvenation procedures was Suzanne Noël (1878–1954), who operated on patients in her own apartment in Paris, in the exclusive sixteenth arrondissement, near the Hotel George V. She trained during World War I, treating facial wounds in the surgical unit of Hippolyte Morestin, associate professor of anatomy at the University of Paris, whose work on facial reconstruction also influenced Harold Gillies when he visited the unit during the war. Noël was the brilliant daughter of a wealthy family, and after the war she dedicated her surgical life until her death, at the age of seventy-four, to the development of aesthetic plastic surgery, especially rejuvenation. Her writings reveal a sympathetic understanding of her patients and make her an excellent guide to the rejuvenation surgery of this era.

Noël's interest in aesthetic plastic surgery was first aroused when she was visited by an actress (thought to be Sarah Bernhardt) who had undergone facial surgery by Charles Conrad Miller in Chicago. Noël wrote:

> In 1921 one of our greatest actresses returned from a glamorous holiday in America and all the news-papers were full of the fact that the diva appeared astonishingly rejuvenated, thanks to an operation carried out on her scalp. This report gave me much to think about. I experimented on my own face to see whether I could, by pinching off the skin of the face in various places and in various directions, get rid of the existing wrinkles. I was astonished at the results of these experiments and set about studying the matter more thoroughly.

Her words vividly convey her excitement as she realised that it might be possible to surgically rejuvenate a face. She asked the actress for details of her operation and was interested to see that Miller had removed a flap of skin from the actress's scalp, from one ear to the other, and had lifted the facial skin to close the wound. This is what we would now call a 'brow lift'; at the time it was enterprising and courageous surgery. It alleviated the actress's frown lines and crow's feet, but of course it would have left the lower part of her face completely unaltered.

Noël started to experiment, first using her own face, then the skin of anaesthetised rabbits, and then, cautiously, that of human patients, starting with very small procedures. As she gained proficiency, developing her own techniques and instruments, she also gained confidence. When she witnessed the effects of her work on the lives of her patients she became a zealous promoter of the surgery. In fact, she believed it to be of great social importance, which was reflected in the title of her 1926 book, *La chirurgie esthétique: son rôle sociale* ('Aesthetic surgery and its social significance').

Many of her patients were working people who either feared or actually suffered loss of work. They lived in an era when discrimination on the basis of age or looks was acceptable, while at the same time there was, in Parisian society, a heightened awareness and emphasis on the body. Noël noted that

> after the armistice in 1918, it was apparent that good living conditions were increasingly difficult to maintain. The greatest impact of this economic downturn was felt by older people, as everywhere youth and beauty took precedence.

If people lost their work, they and their dependants could experience great suffering. One of Noël's patients, who had been a manager in a luxury-goods store before losing her job, fainted while having her stitches removed and was subsequently 'forced to admit that she had not eaten for 48 hours' due to lack of supplies. After being given a meal and support by Noël, the woman, who had previously applied for work in many stores without success, found work the next day, 'in one of the same stores in which she had earlier been most harshly treated'. Noël conducted three more operations on the woman over the next two months, advancing her rejuvenation in small stages—a method she favoured for people who were unable to take time off work.

Noël observed the psychological phenomenon that patients not only looked less tired after surgery but were better able to deal with real tiredness when it occurred. Naturally, this interested her; she concluded that it was the result of the new ease they felt in themselves, relieved of the distress of constantly looking tired. As a result of what she had seen, she considered 'aesthetic surgery to be a true benefactor of humanity, for it enables people of both genders to improve their work opportunities to an extraordinary extent'.

She began to be sought out by those whose 'motivation was the love of beauty and the wish to remain young', including wealthy patients from the aristocracy. She visited surgeons around the world to learn new techniques, crossing the Atlantic fourteen times and, on at least one occasion, operating on fellow passengers en route. In 1928, she was inducted into the Legion of Honour.

Although Noël and other surgeons of the time wrote about the psychological benefits of what they were doing, their work was greeted with suspicion by some. In 1919, surgeon Raymond Passot, who also lived in Paris and later wrote a book on aesthetic surgery, claimed that it was treated with the same suspicion that reconstructive surgery had been met with before the war. As he wrote, reconstructive surgery had finally been accepted, as would aesthetic plastic surgery be—in time. The cycle of acceptance was slow. In the meantime, aesthetic plastic surgery was simply waiting 'in quarantine'.

Noël experienced the same wariness from the surgical fraternity.

> People regarded the concept as ludicrous and scoffed at my reports of it. However, necessity is a hard teacher, and it led my first patients to me. These people had been driven to the edge of despair and regarded aesthetic surgery as their last hope.

As a feminist, suffragette and key mover in the early soroptimist movement (an international society for women in business and the professions), Noël saw rejuvenation as complementary to women's freedom, recognising that it gave opportunities previously denied. 'Is this not a wonderful task that aesthetic surgery performs,' she wrote, 'and does it not deserve to be highly respected and favoured everywhere for its moral worth?' She practised what she preached, having multiple face lifts and eyelid procedures herself, which left her with a smooth, wrinkle-free face.

Many patients were prepared to try whatever could be done. The desire to be rid of the effects of ageing was strong, and having some degree of improvement, even if short-lived or at the expense of a totally natural appearance, was felt to be better than having no improvement at all.

Skin-tightening rejuvenation

Early rejuvenation surgery's superficial 'skin only' simplicity allowed it to be performed in private clinics like Noël's at a time when hospitals were only for sick people. Rejuvenation patients recovered quickly, with immediate visible improvements to their appearance. In fact, it was almost a 'lunchtime lift': Noël recounted operating at six o'clock one evening on a lady who was wearing full evening dress in readiness for a formal dinner later that night. When she arrived at the event after her surgery her friends noted her pleasing appearance and ascribed it to her dress. To disguise their sudden transformation, Noël wrote, 'I advise women to change their hairstyle a little or buy themselves a new hat; this little stratagem suffices to explain away their noticeable beautification'. The photograph of one of her patients sitting up after surgery, wearing a new hat and sipping coffee, is an iconic image of aesthetic plastic surgery.

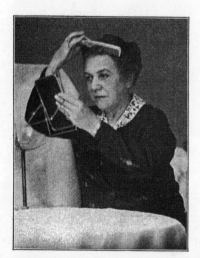 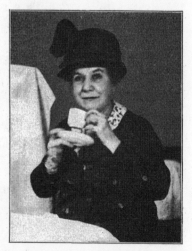

A patient of Dr Suzanne Noël combing her hair after surgery to cover the stitches, after which 'in perfect beauty she enjoys a cup of coffee before returning home to go about her daily activities.'

Charles Willi, characteristically enthusiastic, exclaimed: 'Half an hour for half a new face!' His patients were awake while their face was lifted using local anaesthetic, and they rested at home afterwards merely, Willi said, to aid healing and not because it was considered necessary. It was, he explained, a 'very trifling operation indeed; it leaves no scar at all, and, as carried out, causes no pain'. He compared it with taking a section out of a waistcoat and claimed that it was as harmless as cutting hair or nails, lasting only a few minutes and involving less ordeal than going to a dentist or manicurist.

Seventy years young

At seventy years of age I felt young. I was still working and my face wasn't that lined, but I'd inherited this awful turkey neck, like a huge double chin, which made me look so much older. I hated it—I always had—but I wondered if maybe I was too old to bother getting rid of it. But you care how you look, regardless of your age. And your face and how you feel work together; one is in hand with the other. Sometimes, when I went out, I felt I looked really horrible.

After the surgery I feel this lightness of everything, this whole sense of wellbeing. People say to me all the time, 'You look fantastic,' and that makes me feel great. It's gone way beyond the neck. Everything I do, I do more confidently, because I'm not thinking about looking awful.

The early rejuvenation surgeons took a simple, empirical approach to their surgical procedure. They looked at what appeared to be their patients' main problem—skin laxity—and removed that problem by removing the lax skin. The more laxity there was, the more skin they removed; 'with very advanced wrinkles only significant tightening of the facial skin may obtain a satisfactory result'. The art was to make the excision large enough to provide an effect but not so large that the excess tension would result in a visible scar. The purpose of the procedure was acknowledged in its name, rhytidectomy, from the Greek *rhytis* (wrinkle) and *ectome* (removal of). At its conceptual core was the skin flap, although in a new guise.

Surgeons chose the sites for incisions according to the facial area needing correction as well as their personal preference. They even took their cues from watching what patients did. One surgeon had a patient who before her surgery had pulled the excess skin off her face and held it in place with clips, which she hid in her hair. The surgeon noted the location of her clips and put incisions in those places. Another resourceful patient had done the same with plaster tapes, using them to draw the skin in behind the ears and keep it there, concealed. In most instances, to obtain a result across the entire face, the surgeon made a series of small elliptical incisions around the face and then gently pulled the skin to tighten it. To remove bags under the eyes, a small crescent-shaped piece of skin was cut out just under the lashes; to correct a frown, a small oval piece of skin was removed from above the nose; to remove a double chin, an incision was placed under the chin and hidden in the little cleft there; to improve the neck, a long oval incision was made at the nape of the neck, and the patient was advised to keep their hair long enough to hide the scar.

In time, the use of multiple small incisions gave way to a single continuous incision, from the temple running downwards in front of the ears and curving back behind the lobes. The first 'before and after' face lift photographs were presented in 1919 by Adalbert G Bettman, at the University of Oregon, who used the single incision technique. This early face lift procedure, with its simple reliance on skin tightening, formed the template for face lifts for the next half-century, including the years after World War II, a boom time for aesthetic surgery.

But there were limits to the skin-stretching procedure, largely to do with the skin itself and the role it was asked to play in this sort of face lift. Young skin is elastic, but as it ages the elasticity is lost due to deterioration and weakening of the elastic fibres in the skin. When elastically damaged skin is pulled, a biomechanical change known as 'stress relaxation' results: the collagen fibres that normally crisscross the skin reorientate to become more longitudinal, causing further elongation of the skin over time. This leads to a dilemma for surgeons, because they are trying to achieve a tightening effect in the central part of the face (where the ageing occurs), but this is a long way forward of the incision in front of the ear. So they have to pull the skin tightly across to the incision site and then, to keep the effect, close the incision fairly tightly, which risks a stretched scar. After surgery, the tightened skin becomes even thinner due to the surgical pull on top of the stretch of ageing. The collagen fibres begin to arrange themselves in a parallel pattern, so the face stiffens. The patient may look less saggy immediately after the procedure (as Madame Noël's stories confirm) but in time— usually well before twelve months have passed—their skin will relax. Over the slightly longer term, around four years, much of the earlier benefit will have been lost. Harold Gillies recognised this natural process and recommended that patients routinely had a second tightening, to take up the slack, six months after the first procedure. Suzanne Noël wrote that 'one must nevertheless admit that depreciation of the skin will call for repeated operations', explaining that the skin sags after surgery as a normal bodily process, just as dyed hair grows out, glasses need changing and teeth need to be examined every few years.

After the secondary tightening the collagen fibres remain in their parallel arrangement, so the second face lift, unlike the first, does not have an early relapse, although, of course, the loss of elasticity remains. And this is the reason we associate expressionless faces with repeated surgery of this type. With subsequent procedures, the skin is placed under greater tension and stretched to an unnatural degree. This is when that well-known phenomenon of the 'windswept look' appears, in faces that have been stretched so tightly that the original face has become distorted, sometimes almost beyond recognition. Skin pulling never gives a natural appearance; youthful faces are not youthful because the skin is pulled tightly across them.

Pulling the skin also puts tension on the incision itself, which has to hold the entire result. So the healed incision naturally does what skin will do when it is placed under excessive tension—it stretches and forms a visible scar. Skin-pulling surgery was prone to poor scarring, sometimes producing an obvious unpleasant scar in the hairline or behind, or even worse, in front of the ears. This is anathema to modern aesthetic plastic surgery, in which avoidance of any visible scarring is imperative. Another common effect of skin pulling was the distortion of the earlobe, a complete giveaway. Again, this would be unacceptable in a modern face lift.

There was another, more subtle problem with this procedure: skin tightening's maximum effectiveness occurred close to the incision site, which was, of course, at the edge of the face. But we don't age much at the edge of our face, as it isn't used for communication. Rejuvenation needs to take place in the communication zone, that is, the central column around the eyes and mouth. This took a while for surgeons to realise, and even longer to find a solution for it, so for most of the twentieth century a face lift meant skin tightening.

Noël was pleased that 70 per cent of her patients went to her early for their surgery, when 'a certain tiredness of features has only just become evident' and before 'age has all-too-clearly stamped their features'. But, because the results of skin stretching didn't last long, people began to hold off from having their surgery, often until their faces were looking extremely aged. Nobody wanted to have multiple surgeries by the time they were sixty, so waiting until they were well into their fifties, or even later, made sense. But this made the surgery highly visible to others: one day a person looked like an aged fifty-five-year-old, and the next they looked quite different, with tightened skin and a slightly stretched appearance around the mouth or across the cheeks. There is nothing subtle about that kind of change. It would have been hard to convince people that anything other than surgery had brought about such a transformation.

From the perspective of the twenty-first century, although we can admire the courage and innovations of the early surgeons, it's also painfully clear that their techniques were not based on an understanding of facial ageing, and produced results that were short-lived and overly simplistic, even though they were excellent surgeons. However, while skin tightening did not achieve the subtle or natural look available from today's rejuvenation procedures, practitioners and patients at the time viewed the process with a different attitude from ours. Those surgeons were removing a negative; a completely positive result could not be expected. As Willi said, 'it must merely appear that a youthful spirit has triumphed over tired flesh'.

For many decades the skin-tightening face lift continued to be the only rejuvenation surgery available. Eventually, the loss of natural appearance led some surgeons to question the technique and to look for better procedures. One of these was the renowned plastic surgeon from New York, Gustave Aufricht, who trained with Jacques Joseph in Berlin and was one of the founders of the American Board of Surgery. In 1960, at the Second International Congress of Plastic and Reconstructive Surgery, he presented a technique that added another feature to the traditional skin lift: tightening of the underlying facial layer. It was an early taste of things to come. In 1974, John Burke Tipton, from California, also wrote about tightening the deeper facial tissues in addition to the skin. However, when he tested it by performing two different techniques on the same face—imagine the ethical dilemma!—unexpectedly, he found the results to be similar to the earlier procedure. This was discouraging for those surgeons who had come to believe that this might be a way to improve results. Fortunately, however, one surgeon thinking about facial surgery in the 1970s discovered how to take it to that next level, creating a face lift that overcame the limitations of the skin and producing a result so natural in its appearance that, even today, it continues to impress.

Surgery of the psyche

Before surgery I wondered what was it that lay dormant in me that I wanted to rediscover. And to my surprise, it was my sensuality that had been hung up on a hanger for so many years. I decided I needed to embrace elegance more, embrace rather than fear or be shamed by a little vanity. I would need to make an effort to wardrobe myself to suit who I would now become—but who would this be? It was like trying to imagine the face of the unborn child you are yet to meet.

For a long time I had stopped pondering myself in the mirror because it never seemed to show who I thought I was. I knew I was a younger-looking woman who could still attract eyes and a whistle, not this one who looked like she'd gone without sleep for a week and had had a hard life.

I enjoy people's responses to me now; I enjoy the smiles I more spontaneously receive. Youth is definitely wasted on the young; they are too self-conscious to appreciate and enjoy it freely. I believe my younger looks have given me more power of influence inside and outside of work. I am listened to more and approached more socially. Do I applaud society for valuing youthful looks above experience and wisdom—no, but I'll take it now it's here and be very grateful for it.

13

Finding faces

*I profess to learn and to teach anatomy not from
books but from dissections, not from the tenets
of Philosophers but from the fabric of Nature.*

William Harvey

odern anatomy (a word which comes from a Greek
noun meaning a dissection or cutting up) traditionally has several forms, two of which are classical and
surgical. Classical anatomy teaches the locations of the parts of
the body through description, drawings and photographs in
atlases. Anatomy students study these drawings and then may
make their own while endlessly memorising lines to help them
remember it all. That's what a classical anatomist needs to know,
but for surgeons, classical knowledge is not enough. Surgical
anatomy teaches the application of knowledge gained through
classical anatomy in actual surgical procedures: it is the study of
the body itself, real ligaments, muscles and bones. Knowledge

of both classical anatomy and experience in surgical anatomy are necessary if a surgeon is to be successful. Of course, studying drawings and learning by rote are straightforward enough; gaining experience of anatomy through the dissection of actual bodies, however, has caused difficulties for surgeons through the centuries, as it requires access to cadavers.

People are often surprised that we still don't know everything there is to know about the face. After all, it's quite small, and we've been operating on it for centuries. But the study of anatomy is a classic example of a very human attribute: seeing only what we're looking for. As in so many other areas of life, our knowledge of anatomy has been the product of those who studied it, and those who studied it were themselves the product of the eras in which they lived. For instance, in the twentieth century classical anatomy was developed largely from the work of anatomists in the 1920s and 1930s, whose extensive writings taught subsequent generations. But those decades belonged to the pre-antibiotic era—when a simple scratch could end up being fatal, and once an infection started it couldn't be stopped. So the surgeons studying anatomy had one overriding concern: how to stop people dying from the spread of infection in the soft tissues. If a patient had a facial abscess, surgeons knew that unless it was drained the infection would spread inexorably deeper into the face until it reached an eye or the brain, at which point the patient would die. The question for those surgeons was how they could access the abscess, drain it, stop the spread of infection and save the patient. As a result, almost everything they did, including some stunning works of illustration and publications of anatomy texts, reflected this imperative. Areas of the face that were peripheral and not of clinical importance to them were not researched.

The continued study of anatomy using cadavers is still seen, therefore, as fundamental to surgical life. Cadaver dissection gives surgeons and anatomists information that is otherwise not possible to discover and without which anatomy is completely theoretical. Without a detailed understanding of facial anatomy, it is not possible for facial plastic surgeons to operate at the highest level. This is an example of where classical anatomy has its limits: a facial surgeon needs to know not just that the facial nerve is 'somewhere in this area'; they should know precisely where it is and how to find and isolate it before proceeding with the surgery. It is only through experience of the elements themselves that it is possible to truly know the different layers of the face, the relationships between its structures, how they connect to each other and where the landmarks are. In order to develop improved techniques and complex procedures, access is needed to a human face so that detailed anatomy can be defined and new surgery tested to see how it works anatomically. This can't be done without cadavers.

Accessing cadavers

Surgeons try to conduct or observe cadaver dissection whenever possible—for example, in return for teaching at a university or as part of a workshop. But entry is extremely limited. Some universities have programs through which people can bequeath their body to anatomical research specifically for authorised research projects and not for surgical training, although ready access to this material requires formal affiliation with a university department. Making matters more difficult for facial surgeons, not any cadaver will do for the detailed needs of facial surgery. The face must be 'fresh', which in most cases means frozen and thawed out the night before work begins. Cadaver material that has been embalmed in formalin for long-term keeping, while useful for teaching medical students, is not suitable for facial surgeons, as the tissues become dried out and brown, and are not sufficiently lifelike or useful for surgical guidance.

Mortuary material—bodies on which post-mortems have been carried out—is protected by law in most countries, including Australia. This ensures the purpose of the dissection is specifically about defining the cause of death. Before researchers or surgeons can be granted access to such cadavers, approval is required from both an ethics committee—only possible for research and not for surgical training—and the family, which means that these bodies are rarely available, and when they are it's usually at short notice and during odd hours. Working with a dead body deep in a morgue is a long way from the glamorous life so often attributed to plastic surgeons. For this type of dissection surgeons are not permitted to make fresh incisions but have to use those created during the post-mortem, to ensure that no further damage is done to the body. Enormous respect is given to the body, and great care is taken of it. There is always an emotional dimension to operating on dead people, and it raises questions about the sanctity of life—and the need to keep people whole even in death—which is fundamental to certain religions.

Surgeons can pay to attend cadaver dissection workshops—which are conducted in several countries, such as Austria, Thailand, the United States and Australia—that focus on specific parts of the face. These courses use heads of cadavers that are purchased and shipped in as part of an extensive—and legal—trade in cadaver materials. Most of these seem to travel via the United States. Legal cadaver parts come with a signficiant amount of paperwork in order to verify their source, to ensure against transmissible diseases such as HIV and hepatitis, and to certify that they have been managed with the appropriate respect. A legally purchased cadaver head can cost around $3000, which demonstrates the need for regulation in such a potentially lucrative area, and there are considerable on-costs to pay for their special care in anatomy departments and their ultimate disposal.

A recent development that diminishes the need for cadavers is live surgical demonstrations. At many of today's surgical conferences, a surgeon is invited to perform the operation for which they are renowned in front of cameras that transmit live images to a conference room where hundreds of other surgeons can observe the action. The close-up capability of the television camera lens allows the audience to see the procedure in greater detail than the surgeon actually performing the operation. The audience can also hear the surgeon explaining their work as they operate and can ask questions through a moderator, not unlike during dissections in the early days of the anatomical theatres in Bologna and Padua, when the anatomy professor would demonstrate and reply to questions from his audience. Today, two or more operating theatres are often used simultaneously, sparing the audience the tedious parts of the surgery—much surgery is fairly tedious—and allowing the moderator to switch views as the action warrants. It is instructive to see surgical judgement in action and to watch how an expert handles a difficult part of an operation.

Live surgical demonstrations and edited surgical videos are an excellent way of advancing the skills of established surgeons, but the need for traditional cadaver dissection remains to this day as advances in anatomical understanding directly relate to improvements in surgical procedures, allowing them to be understood in a three-dimensional way and in relation to adjacent vital structures within the body. This is not something to be learnt in the operating theatre at the patient's expense.

14

The anatomy of ageing

The countenance is the portrait of the soul,
and the eyes mark its intentions.

Cicero

The plastic surgeon who brought about the great change in face lift techniques was Tord Skoog (1915–1977). He trained at Sweden's Uppsala University, and also with Gillies and McIndoe in England, and became accomplished in many facets of reconstructive plastic surgery. Before his major breakthrough he had already published his techniques for several other surgical problems, including reduction mammoplasty, correction of Dupuytren's contracture of the hand (which causes fingers to be permanently bent down towards the palm) and cleft lip repair. The Tord Skoog Society developed around him, an international gathering of elite thinkers, bright young surgeons who benefited from a high-level exchange of ideas. When Skoog turned his rigorous thinking to face lift surgery, a new era began. By the end of the 1970s face lift procedures and the thinking underlying them were radically different from what they had been only ten years earlier.

It began in 1969, when Skoog gave a presentation at the annual congress of the American Society of Plastic Surgeons entitled 'Useful Techniques in Facelifting', which was received with some astonishment by the surgeons who heard it. In Skoog, the field of anatomy had found an interested thinker asking questions that went beyond simply focusing on what he needed to know. (He was rare in his field: as we have seen, anatomy has a history of people seeing only what they are looking for.) Unlike almost everyone else, Skoog did not focus on the obvious loose skin of ageing, but thought about it at a more fundamental level. He questioned *why* the skin's appearance changed over time and what was causing the laxity and found the reason in the fibrous support layer *beneath* the skin, known as the superficial fascia. His claim was quite startling: that the laxity responsible for facial ageing occurs below the surface of the skin, not in the skin itself.

Other experts were sceptical. After all, anyone could tell just by looking at older people that it was their skin that was loose; it was obvious that ageing created the appearance of excess skin. If the skin were disregarded, how could a proper rejuvenation be achieved? (It's worth remembering that in those days, every face lift patient was old, so loose skin was the obvious feature of their ageing.)

But then in 1974 came Skoog's magnificent textbook, *Plastic Surgery: New methods and refinements*, published simultaneously in Swedish, English, Japanese, Italian and Spanish. It contained a separate chapter covering each of his operations, including one on his face lift technique. The procedure was superbly illustrated with intraoperative photographs and included just one set of before and after photographs. But this one result was remarkable, quite beyond anything previously achieved or even imagined. In fact, it still rates today as an outstanding result. At this point, Skoog began to win converts to his way of thinking.

Two years later, in 1976, a seminal article appeared in the most prestigious journal of plastic surgery, *Plastic and Reconstructive Surgery*, written by French surgeons Vladimir Mitz and Martine Peyronie, in which a new name was introduced for Skoog's superficial fascia—the 'superficial muscular aponeurotic system', commonly known by the acronym SMAS—and changed aesthetic plastic surgery forever. It provided another example of breaking through the constrained thinking of the past, of looking at anatomy with a questioning mind. From now on, all thinking about the face lift increasingly involved the SMAS, although our progress towards new procedures was to take many years.

The SMAS

Inside the human body there are internal, or visceral, muscles, associated with the organs, and there are skeletal muscles, which move the bones. They are all located beneath the deep fascia, which is the thin but strong fibrous layer of tissue that surrounds all the muscles and bones of the body. Imagine a skinned rabbit lying in a butcher's display: despite the lack of fur and skin you can see that it's a rabbit. All the muscles and bones are held together in a neat rabbity shape by a sinewy, slightly greyish sack covering the entire body, so the rabbit doesn't fall to pieces when the skin is removed. This outer holding layer is the deep fascia. If we were to replace the skin over the deep fascia, we would also replace the subcutaneous ('beneath the skin') tissue, which is called the superficial fascia and is used mainly for fat storage. The human body, just like that rabbit, has outer layers consisting of skin and superficial fascia, except in one area: the face.

In the human face, there are two additional layers of tissue, and these are necessary to allow movement of the face. The first of these is the SMAS, which is located *within* the superficial fascia and consists of muscles that move the outer layers—creating facial expressions—as well as the fibrous tissue that surrounds and connects those muscles. The SMAS can be imagined as a tough, elastic web that covers the whole face and holds those muscles in place. The three uppermost facial layers—skin, superficial fascia and SMAS—are fused together, which allows them to move as one composite unit, gliding over the deeper layers. The second extra layer, the loose areolar, lies directly beneath the top three layers and mainly consists of loose connective tissue that acts as a gliding plane. Its gliding ability is critical to facial expression, because if the outer three layers were not able to move over the deeper layers, the human face would be a rigid mask, as expressionless as that of a fish. If you place your hand on your forehead and then raise and lower your eyebrows, you can feel the glide.

The human face has two different layers of muscles. We have just discussed the first, which forms part of the SMAS, and to which we will return shortly. The second muscle layer, which is of less importance to our discussion of the face lift, is only on the side of the face, deeper in beneath the soft tissue and deep fascia. It forms the powerful muscles of mastication, which work the lower jaw. If you place a finger on each cheek in front of the ear, then clench and unclench your jaw, you can feel the first of these muscles—called the masseters—tighten. Gradually move your fingers forwards as you keep clenching the jaw and you will eventually come to the front edge of the muscles. Repeat the jaw clenching with your fingers placed on your temples, and you'll feel the contraction of the second muscle of mastication—the temporalis.

The facial layers

Imagine that you have sliced through the soft tissue of the face as far as the deep fascia and are looking at it with the sliced edge towards you. There are five layers, which are, starting with the outermost layer:

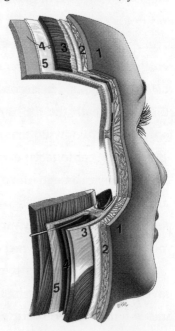

1 skin
2 superficial fascia: the fatty layer, also known as the subcutaneous layer
3 SMAS: fibrous tissue and muscle forming one layer, also known as the aponeurotic fascia
4 loose areolar: the gliding pane
5 deep fascia: a thin layer of dense connective tissue

As we have seen, the SMAS muscle layer is quite different, and the reason is that it's derived from the primitive platysma, discussed in chapter 1. It is just below the skin, and moves the outer layers of facial tissue, including the skin. Lower-order species have more primitive versions of the SMAS muscles in the outer facial layers and their function is to move the soft tissues that overlie the bony cavities—for example, to open and close the eyes and mouth. The twitching of a dog's nose shows this layer of muscle in use around the nasal cavity. The muscles are linked to the nervous system, which has an instantaneous 'automatic function' to protect the individual from danger. When a horse flares its nostrils and raises its ears, biologically, this is to help breathing and hearing as part of the 'fight or flight' reflex, geared to enhance performance in a critical moment for survival. In humans, however, the function of the outer layer of muscles in the nose and ears has reduced over time, while additional movement has evolved in the muscles of the eyes and mouth—the communication zone—which are involved in the additional 'new' functions of expression and speech.

The discovery that it is the deep layers of the face, and not just the skin, which become lax with age was fundamental to improvements in facial rejuvenation surgery. It meant that focusing on the skin alone was not enough. Of course, the skin does age, but it only *adds* to the look of age; it doesn't create it. Badly aged skin on a thirty-year-old wouldn't make that person look sixty; they would look like a younger person with severely damaged skin. A person begins to look old only once the deeper layers of the face have become lax. So, while staying out of the sun in youth helps to reduce sun damage and skin ageing, the deeper structural changes of age continue regardless, and facial ageing still appears. Think of the ageing face of famous figures who have typically avoided the sun, such as Queen Elizabeth II.

After the description of the SMAS, plastic surgeons started to think differently about the sequence of ageing and planned their procedures differently as a result. Skin laxity, the previous focus of face lift surgery, became secondary to laxity in the SMAS. Any correction of ageing had to include correction of laxity in the SMAS layer, as this was the source of the skin laxity. Surgeons found that rejuvenating the SMAS by operating directly on that layer restored the face to a more natural youthful shape, after which the skin could simply be draped over the rejuvenated layer without the need for any pressure, pulling or tightening. This, in turn, eliminated the many problems that had been caused by stretching the skin, especially scarring at the sites of the incisions. By correcting ageing at its source, it seemed that a natural and lasting rejuvenation could finally be achieved.

The description of the SMAS was a true eureka moment in facial anatomy, completely revising our understanding of how the human face functions.

The SMAS face lift

It was one thing to know about the SMAS but quite another to use it surgically for rejuvenation. Plastic surgeons were keen to develop a procedure that would correct the sagging and deep grooves in the skin caused by laxity of the SMAS, thereby rejuvenating facial shape. It was also believed that the results would be longer lasting than those of the skin-tightening procedure, allowing patients to have surgery earlier and then simply appear to age well in the future. This would be a wonderful step forward, and the thinking was correct, but it actually took another twenty years of development to achieve what was hoped for.

Nevertheless, many surgeons started to tighten the SMAS as part of their face lift procedure. Most did a conventional skin lift first and then elevated the SMAS as a separate layer for a short distance from the incision in front of the ear. Some were happy with the results. They felt that the outcomes were better and the scars in front of the ears were definitely improved. Their patients also seemed to be pleased with the surgery.

But the reality was there were no clear directions for surgeons. For many surgeons the improvement wasn't significant enough and they gave up on the technique, feeling that the benefits didn't compensate for the extra time that the SMAS surgery took.

Also, a new complication appeared with alarming frequency—weakness of an area of the facial muscles, particularly the lower lip on one side or weak eyelid closure, due to damage to branches of the important facial nerve. We have all seen newsreaders on television looking well but with a visible lip weakness. The damage occurred because the nerve branches are located just beneath the SMAS and spread out across the face from close to the ears, in the fourth layer of facial tissue. Operating to lift the SMAS brought surgeons into proximity with these nerve branches, which could be stretched, bruised or, worse still, accidently cut. Most of these injuries were transient, but the surgeon and patient would not know if the damage was temporary or permanent until weeks later, when recovery of the muscle function appeared or failed to appear.

It seemed as though the answer to facial ageing had been found, but the practical applications of that knowledge for facial rejuvenation remained elusive.

Gradually, however, answers emerged. It became apparent that the failure to achieve a major improvement was due to the surgery being performed on the least important part of the face, the outer section between the ear and outer cheek. It was realised that ageing occurs in the communication zone, the part of the face that is constantly moving and that other people focus on; that is, the central part, which includes the eyes, the inner cheek and the mouth. The sides of the face, by contrast, are relatively static and don't add much to our communication, nor do they age significantly. But because the incisions were placed at the ears, the area closest to the ears received the most correction, so the aesthetic improvement was not generally noticeable. (Today, this early SMAS face lift procedure is still performed by some surgeons and is called the S lift, or the mini SMAS lift, and it is promoted as being a quicker, simpler alternative to the full SMAS lift. This is true, but it's at the expense of not focusing on the important central part of the face.)

In order to achieve satisfactory results in the communication zone, the SMAS needed more than this simple tightening from the sides. The surgeon had to work their way—under the skin, of course—from the incisions close to the ears into the centre of the face to work on the SMAS where the most ageing had occurred, in order to resuspend the SMAS on the bones. But the further the surgeon ventured towards the central part of the face, the greater the risk of damage to the facial nerve branches. Surgeons didn't even know the precise locations of the nerve branches; while they had been mapped in classical anatomy, the details needed for safe surgery were simply not available. Fear of the consequences of damaging the nerve, which include permanent facial paralysis, was so profound that most surgeons continued to stay at the edges of the face, leaving untouched the exact points where they most needed to go.

In 1980, the American surgeons Mark Lemmon, a senior surgeon familiar with Tord Skoog's operation, and Sam Hamra in Dallas, Texas, published their experience in performing close to five hundred and eighty SMAS face lifts over five years. Hamra then pushed forwards and developed his own operations. His introduction of the term 'deep plane' in 1990 (to describe the fourth layer glide plane beneath the SMAS) was the key to widespread awareness of the SMAS procedure among plastic surgeons.

Hamra's development gave clear guidance on the importance of operating in the deep plane. The operation evolved further, becoming the composite face lift by 1992, and his book *Composite Rhytidectomy* (1993) covered many technical details of the procedure, including the direction that the SMAS should be fixed to the firm tissue in front of the top of the ear with 'exceptional tension'. Hamra was an excellent surgeon, although his published work lacked the specific anatomical details needed to fully explain his operation. The results of his surgery looked somewhat overcorrected, but did avoid the unpopular 'windswept' look.

At the same time, John Owsley Jr, a distinguished surgeon in San Francisco, California, was contributing to face lift developments, but with a less maverick approach, in that his published articles included the anatomical basis for his SMAS platysma surgery. Mitz and Peyronie had advised—in their 1974 paper on the SMAS—that surgeons should not operate forward of the parotid gland, due to the real risk of damage to the facial nerves. But Hamra and Owsley did exactly that, taking their operations forward of the parotid gland, and finally gaining the results we had been waiting for—despite venturing into tiger country as far as potential nerve risk was concerned.

Hamra and Owsley, like Skoog before them, were pioneering surgeons, at a time when a reliable anatomical map of the facial nerve was still lacking.

Facial ligaments

Tord Skoog's discovery of the SMAS raised many further questions. For example, *how* did the SMAS age, and what caused its gradual laxity in certain areas? Thirteen years after Skoog's description of the SMAS, in 1989, another classic contribution to our understanding of facial ageing was published by plastic surgeon David Furnas, who worked in Irvine, California, although he also dedicated a large part of his life to operating on the indigenous peoples of East Africa. He developed a meticulous face lift technique using high-power magnification, which reputedly took up to fourteen hours—immensely long for a face lift procedure. During the surgery, thanks to the magnification and Furnas's careful technique, he was able to see something that had not been noticed by others: in certain areas of the face there is a stronger adherence of the superficial fascia (the second layer of facial tissue) to the outer surface of the SMAS (the third layer) than in other areas. Following cadaver dissections in which he mapped the different sections, he was able to describe a new element of facial anatomy: facial ligaments, also called the retaining ligaments of the face.

Facial movement is a type of balancing act. As well as movement, the face needs stability. We don't want our lower eyelids to be pulled down every time we open our mouth, or our cheeks to be so loose that we need to lift them up to get food into our mouth. The forces that allow mobility and the forces that govern stability need to be in balance. Anatomically,

Furnas discovered, this balance is held between the muscles, which create movement, and the ligaments, which are like tiny stitches, some large and strong and others small, which hold all the soft tissue onto the bones of the face. It's quite an ask, and there are consequences to all this balancing. When as a young person we tip our face down to look at the floor, the facial soft tissues don't sag away from the bones. As we age, however, there is greater looseness when we lower our head: the ligaments, as throughout the rest of the ageing body, have become weaker and stretched a bit, meaning that they give way more to the pull of gravity. When the ligaments of the face become lax in this way, the muscles of the SMAS are held less tightly onto the facial bones, and this is what causes the ageing of the SMAS. The wonderful mobility of our face, the very element that gives life to our appearance, predisposes it to ageing.

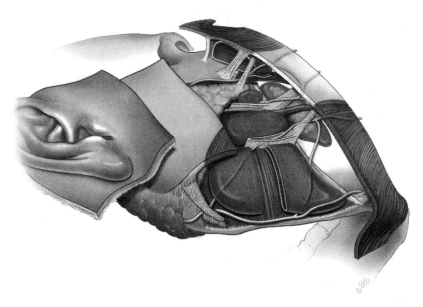

Facial ligaments are tree-like structures that connect the superficial fascia (layers 1–3) to the underlying bone.

Shrinking bones

The final jigsaw piece in the anatomy of ageing was added in 2001 with the discovery that as we age some of our facial bones shrink. In fact, this shrinkage is so significant that we can virtually tell the age of a person by the state of their bones.

The human skull, which provides the frame on which our face is built, is composed largely of cavities: the big empty spaces for the eyes and mouth. These leave only a small area of bone around and between them to 'prop up' the face, and it is to this bone that the muscles and ligaments are attached, which in turn hold the rest of the face in place. As this small support area of bone diminishes through shrinkage, so does the amount of support it can provide.

In some people, the maxillae (the inner cheek bones), which run down from under each eye, along the side of the nose to the upper teeth, become so thin they are almost translucent, something like an eggshell. This may help explain why some people snore more as they get older: the support given to their nose by the cheekbones has decreased, allowing the soft tissues to collapse into the nasal passages and leading to decreased space for air to flow through. It also provides an explanation as to why the nose droops as we age: it has lost some of its support. Studies using computerised tomography (CT) scans have shown that the angle of the maxillae changes with age, flattening by as much as ten degrees between youth and old age. This is highly significant for facial ageing. As the maxillae flatten, the angle of the cheekbones from the eyes down also flattens—their projection can actually be reduced by up to six millimetres in women and more in men.

These discoveries showed that the complete opposite of what anatomists and plastic surgeons used to believe was actually true: it was once thought that the facial skeleton enlarged with age, with the sole exception of the jawbone if a person lost their teeth. The thinking at the time was that if a person had retained their teeth the plastic surgeon didn't need to look at their skeleton, as this meant they'd also retained their bone structure.

Our new awareness that areas of the facial skeleton actually shrink as we age has provided an important insight into the overall ageing of the human face. It demonstrates that facial tissues actually lose support from the bone structure over time and this, as well as the structural change itself brought about by bone loss, has to be factored into our thinking in rejuvenation surgery.

Facial spaces

Put together shrinkage in the facial bones, stretching of the liga-ments that attach to the bones and laxity in the SMAS, and the whole face is affected: its overall shape changes, the relation-ships between the different parts are altered. Together there is reduced tightness of the tissues that allows more movement to occur from muscle contraction (there is more movement in the smile of an older person than a younger person) and the result is 'crowding' beneath the skin, which causes the bulges, grooves and lines on the overlying skin—replacing the smooth, uninterrupted surface of a young face.

It's a bit like a country road that deteriorates after rain, when the sinking substructure causes ripples and hollows on the surface above. But with a face we know exactly where these hollows will occur, based on the attachment of the ligaments beneath.

In order to achieve the best possible rejuvenation, surgeons needed to take up the laxity in the SMAS, ideally by tightening the facial ligaments to 'rehang' the SMAS onto the facial bones, all in the central zone of the face, and all the while avoiding the facial nerve branches. To make this journey through the anatomy of the face, surgeons needed a 'safe passage' beneath the SMAS, to safely access the central zone from the remote incisions at the sides. Imagine entering a house and having to make your way to a central room either through a series of obstruction-laden tunnels or through another, empty room. This 'room' was discovered in 2001 in the fourth layer of the facial tissue directly over the outer cheek bone, and named the prezygomatic space.

Ageing changes

The junction between the soft tissue of the lower eyelid and that of the cheek provides a useful example of how facial ageing works. In a young person there is a smooth expanse of skin that flows evenly from the lower eyelid across to the cheekbone. In an older person the segments of the junction are revealed, with a drooping bulge below the eye and loss of the attractive smoothness. This shows that the soft tissue of the cheek, which used to sit high up over the cheekbone, has dropped slightly, due to a small but critical loss of bone in this area, and this has placed additional strain on the ligament supporting the upper cheek, which has yielded slightly so that it no longer supports the cheek tissue as effectively as it did in youth. The combination of the descent of the cheek tissue and the increased droop of the lower lid, which descends a few millimetres below the bony rim of the cavity, completely changes the configuration from young and fresh-looking to tired-looking.

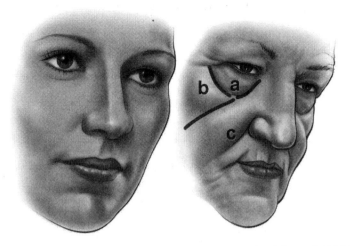

Ageing changes of the mid cheek. A. lid bag, B. malar mound and C. nasolabial fold

This small area under the eye is not what comes to mind for most people when they think of facial ageing. But once you start to really look at faces and notice the change in that area between youth and age, its role in the appearance of ageing becomes obvious.

One week, in 2001, Dr Ashad Muzzafar, resident in plastic surgery at the University of Texas, Southwestern Medical School, and I pored over heads in Dallas, dissecting, discussing and exploring the inner layers of the face. Our interest was in the relationship of the facial nerve to the ligaments in the upper cheek, but after three days we suddenly sensed that a functional space might exist in this area of the face. Our mental framework changed and made allowance for the possibility of its existence. It was the necessary change of mindset: we found a space in the soft tissues in the next day's dissection. We were as exhilarated as explorers finding new land. On the plane back home I knew we'd found the key to understanding the area. It was an amazing feeling.

Subsequently, with spaces in mind, further cadaver research revealed yet another series lower in the cheeks, which were called the premasseter spaces.

If we return to the room analogy regarding facial spaces, the ceiling is the facial muscle, and the floor is layer five in the facial tissue—the deep fascia. There are soft columns inside the rooms, which provide safe housing for the facial nerve branches, just as boxing is used to conceal and protect wiring and plumbing in a house. It was almost as if the space had been made for surgical access, with all the vital structures carefully contained in the columns, allowing surgeons to safely isolate and work around them. Before this discovery, it had been known that it was easier to operate under the SMAS in certain areas, but we didn't know why. No existing work of anatomy described facial spaces or even speculated that they might exist.

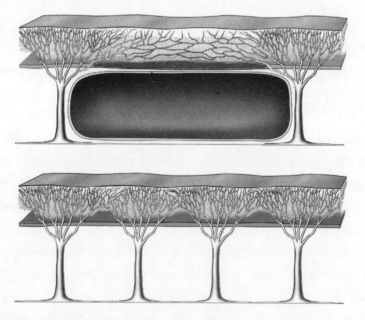

Facial spaces, located under the SMAS, allow a safe surgical passage between the tree-like ligaments.

The discovery that there are facial spaces in the cheeks made the complete SMAS face lift procedure possible by reducing concerns about possible nerve damage. Surgeons could access the communication zone in a safer and more predictable manner, and without bleeding, as there are no vessels or nerves in the spaces. It also helped surgeons to focus on parts of the face that, when adjusted, give a disproportionate benefit to the overall look, such as the corner of the mouth and the jowls.

Many variations of the SMAS technique are in use today and surgeons naturally tend to favour their own techniques. That's why we have conferences, to share our knowledge and ideas. For medical practitioners who operate on the face but lack proper surgical training, the SMAS techniques are far too advanced, leaving them with no option but to continue directing their patients towards the old skin-tightening procedure.

But for surgeons who have the necessary knowledge and skill to perform the full SMAS face lift, the developments mean that they can at last give results in line with their understanding of the SMAS and the way in which it ages. More than ever before, quality facial rejuvenation has become a complex blend of anatomical knowledge, surgical skill, aesthetic judgement and individual assessment. Surgeons are no longer confined to the one-size-fits-all approach of skin tightening, and facial rejuvenation has developed into a satisfying procedure that helps people to subtly and imperceptibly look better as they age.

15

Neck rejuvenation and facial enhancement

The doctor succeeds in his mission when he is able to help, even with bodily alterations that are no illness.

Emil Meirowsky

The neck is a subject all of its own. An ugly neck, and there are surprisingly a lot of them about, can completely detract from an otherwise attractive face. This happens at any age, but for most people the neck is associated with ageing. Nora Ephron won many smiles when she called her book of essays on life and ageing *I Feel Bad About My Neck*. So do many people. I can recall standing beside a very accomplished plastic surgeon in the early 1970s as he told a patient, 'we can fix your cheeks, but not your neck.' Fortunately, that is no longer the case.

Neck rejuvenation

Some people develop greater ageing on the neck than on the face itself, so neck rejuvenation is a subject of considerable importance. It used to be said that the neck was the one place that could not be satisfactorily improved by aesthetic plastic surgery. Even though surgeons tightened the skin of the neck as part of a face lift, failure to improve the full neck was common, and the large amount of early skin relapse was often so great that the patient and indeed the surgeon were extremely disappointed, especially if it was the neck that had been the focus of a major improvement.

The situation changed in 1974, before the emergence of SMAS surgery on the face, with the appearance of an article by José Guerrero-Santos et al. about contouring the neck using a novel approach: shaping the underlying platysma muscle layer as well as removing excess subcutaneous fat. This transformed patients' necks in what seemed to be a miraculous way. The writers of the article had realised that the contour improvement had to take place in the support layer rather than in the skin above it; tightening the skin alone could not achieve the same results. The principles underlying this procedure were, of course, the same as those of the later SMAS face lift. Removal of subcutaneous fat from the neck through a horizontal incision in the crease under the chin had been presented a few years earlier as effective and safe, but it took the addition of the deeper platysma contouring to convincingly correct ageing in the neck.

Plastic surgeon Bruce Connell, in Orange County, south of Los Angeles, continued to develop platysma surgery, giving important presentations and publishing key articles to the point that the procedure became synonymous with his name.

His meticulous and aesthetic approach raised the standard for undetectable aesthetic surgery, and this had a huge influence on the younger generation of aesthetic plastic surgeons while giving greater credibility to platysma—and later, by extension, SMAS—surgery. Much longer operating times were required, sometimes double the time taken for a straightforward skin lift, but it was clear from Connell's results that the end justified the means. Connell was also an interesting example of an aspect of aesthetic plastic surgery that is not found in other fields: the possibility for a private practitioner to have a profoundly important worldwide influence. Connell didn't work in a renowned institution, and his contribution was practical rather than academic or scientific.

There's something fascinating about the fact that rejuvenation surgery and the ancient platysma muscle, which played such a key role in the early development of the face, should intersect in such an influential way in the late twentieth century in Orange County. The development of a technique for the neck was such an amazing step forward in rejuvenation surgery that for many years the neck actually became the focus of new face lift techniques, especially in the United States. In fact, so dramatic were the changes possible that many necks were overdone and unnaturally sculpted. More was not always better: surgeons had to harness the power of the technique to achieve the aesthetic results requested.

The improvements continued. Liposuction, introduced in the 1980s, is beneficial for most necks as a simple alternative to the open surgical removal of fat that was performed previously. In young people with fat necks, liposuction alone can be remarkably effective, and the fat does not come back. But if the neck skin is already loose, liposuction will loosen it more, so a skin-tightening procedure needs to be performed at the same time. Neck rejuvenation remains a key topic at plastic surgery conferences today. Some patients are born with an overly thick neck, lacking definition from chin to throat. This is an anatomical structure where the muscles of the floor of the mouth go lower into the neck than normal and, unfortunately, this cannot be improved by surgery. Others, who have a heavy bulge at the sides of the neck, can be assisted by the removal of the outer part of the submandibullar salivary glands, which is difficult surgery and has the theoretical risk of leaving the patient with a dry mouth. In my experience this is a successful procedure for these patients and does not leave a dry mouth, but it does raise the question of how far we are justified in operating to improve appearance. Does it extend to the removal of part of the body's organ system?

Bone enhancement

Bill Little, a renowned plastic surgeon from Washington, DC, brought an artist's perspective to facial rejuvenation and the pleasing lines of the face in a classic paper published in 2000. He claimed that the only flat part of the face should be under the chin, and that the shape of the cheek, looking at it from an oblique angle, should be like an ogee curve. This term, from architecture, describes a double curve shaped like a flattened S, formed from a convex line joined to a concave line. In other words, flat cheeks are not as attractive as full cheeks, and ageing takes away some of the desirable cheek volume.

In faces in which this bone projection is lacking—through being too flat or through significant shrinkage in some areas— earlier onset of ageing or more extreme facial ageing occurs.

Most of us have areas of facial weakness, or sunken bone structure, and it will be in those places that ageing shows up first.
For example, flatness of the bones under the eyes—a classic
problem— leads to premature and exaggerated lower lid bags,
with sagging of the cheek ligaments.

People who are blessed with a 'good' bone structure fare
better than other people when it comes to ageing. Well-formed
cheekbones and a strong forehead and jawline slow the appearance of ageing because they give extra support to the ligaments
and muscles, holding them in place and thereby helping to resist
sagging. Conversely, those with poor bone structure develop
laxity at a younger age. It is often said that people with Asian
backgrounds age well, and research has shown that people of
Asian descent have a prominent bone structure, which slows
the shrinking of the bones, and wideness across the cheekbones,
which provides more room for the tissues to rest upon, enabling
the face to maintain its attractive youthful shape even as ageing
changes occur.

Since the discovery of the important role played by the
skeleton in facial ageing, bone enhancement using implants has
become an integral component in facial rejuvenation surgery.
A welcome benefit of bone enhancement is that adding bone-
substitute mass in the right places and in the right ways can
slow the rate of ageing on the face, because of the better support
provided to the soft tissues.

Implants are used either to improve the skeleton of a
younger person whose face may be lacking in certain key areas
or to build up areas from which bone has been lost in an ageing
face. The most common sites for this are the cheekbones, the
chin and along the jaw. But augmenting a facial skeleton has to
be done subtly and aesthetically. Like all procedures, it is prone

to overuse or poor use, or to being considered a quick solution. It is frequently misjudged, and we have all seen celebrities whose exaggerated cheekbones and jaws bear no relation to the structure of the rest of their face.

Bone enhancement is not always the quick solution people hope for. As an example, if a face is showing clear signs of ageing and a surgeon uses just bone enhancement to build up the cheekbones, the patient will have larger cheekbones—with sagging tissues hanging beneath them. That's not a youthful look; in fact, it's not a natural look at all. In youth the cheekbone *is* more defined, but it also has a good amount of soft tissue overlying it, giving the effect of roundness. I learnt this lesson early on, with a thirty-eight-year-old patient who practised interior design and therefore had a good eye for detail. He requested cheek implants. Technically, the surgery went well, but the result was not as shapely as we had expected. The reason was that I had underestimated the amount of existing tissue laxity. In other words, the horse had already bolted. It took a later face lift over the implants to tighten the cheek tissue sufficiently to obtain the smooth, shapely, more defined cheeks he wanted. To truly replicate the cheekbones of youth, soft tissue must be lifted back to the more youthful position, so the bones and the tissue *together* create soft, attractive cheeks. Of course, this is considerably more complex than simply adding an implant, but in many cases it's what needs to be done.

The original cheek implants were small oval buttons of silicone, designed to exaggerate the oblique part of the cheek. Later, a teardrop shape was used for the front of the cheek. The implants were initially placed into the soft tissue, but it was found that after a while the tissue over the implants thinned, which created an exaggerated bulge under the skin. After some controversy, the implants were placed directly on the bone surface. Another limitation was that the implants came in pre-formed factory-made sizes ordered from a catalogue, and they weren't always suitable for the purpose. Commonly, they didn't fit the bone surface perfectly, leaving a small hollow space that filled with fluid and created a potential site of infection.

Silicone implants are still widely used, but many surgeons prefer porous polyethylene implants. These are rigid, in contrast to the solid but soft silicone, but have pores that allow the tissues to grow right into them. The implants are more difficult to work with and need to be securely fixed to the underlying bones with small titanium screws.

Personally, I prefer hydroxyapatite, a natural material derived from coral, which is almost identical to bone in chemical composition and its porous structure. It comes in a granular form (something like coarse sand) and is formed to a putty-like consistency in surgery, then placed on the bone and formed to the individual requirement of the patient. Within a day it fuses to the bone and then sets in that position, creating a permanent structure to build an improved shape or restore what has been lost through bone shrinkage. I include hydroxyapatite as part of most rejuvenation procedures, as just a tiny amount of enhancement in the right place gives a disproportionately beneficial result. When done properly, with careful judgement, it is not noticed by other people, as the patient simply moves from a negative to a normal appearance.

The most common bone enhancement approach is fat injections. These are simple to perform, and a moderate amount of fat readily compensates for small areas of bone shrinkage. But if a larger area requires correction, the fat, being soft, inherently lacks the structure necessary to provide the bone-like definition that is the foundation of an attractive facial shape.

Our knowledge about the role of bone shrinkage in facial ageing is recent and is slowly being appreciated for its importance. The idea would have astonished the early practitioners in aesthetic surgery. It would have been inconceivable to them that the invisible skeleton—and the deeper tissues—were more important than the highly visible skin.

Fat injections

Replacement of fat on the face to increase volume using the patient's own fat is an important aspect of facial rejuvenation, but it isn't as straightforward as it may sound. The overuse of fat injections has led to a common phenomenon—the 'pillow-faced' look—faces that are as swollen and puffy as a body that is carrying too much fat. This can create an amorphous look in which patients risk losing their facial identity, because fat faces tend to look the same. Through the excessive desire to reduce the appearance of wrinkles and lines much distinctiveness is lost, including proportion and individuality.

However, injecting small amounts of fat can be a very useful solution when used with good aesthetic judgement or to complete the effect of surgery, such as gently plumping up the area around the eyes after rejuvenation surgery to overcome a gaunt look and to create an attractive, softer appearance. Young people naturally have plumpness in the upper lid, so giving a subtle volume to this area can be helpful. It is not enough simply to remove laxity in the area; the result can be overly gaunt, and it's not desirable to see into the crease above the eye. In youth that rarely happens; in fact, youthful upper lids can be quite full.

An extremely small amount of fat is required. The procedure moves living cells from one part of the body to another, where they take up residence with a blood supply. Once the fat has gained a blood supply, it survives permanently. However, the fat cells continue to behave as fat, so if, following a fat injection, a patient puts on weight, the fat transferred to the face will behave just like fat from the abdomen, where it came from. I once had a very thin patient with gaunt, deep-set eyes, who looked greatly improved with the introduction of a little fat. However, the patient later put on weight, the fat cells became enlarged, and I ended up taking out more fat than I had originally put in.

Vaseline and paraffin wax

Aesthetic facial injections are not a new phenomenon. They are mentioned in historical records as early as 1900, when Vaseline was used to correct facial defects. But it was quickly found to be unsuitable, due to localised reactions and even serious complications leading to death.

The next product tried was low-melting-point paraffin wax, which was popular for about twenty years. It was used, for instance, on the bridge of the nose, to fill in or reshape a deformity. It became so popular that the injecting of paraffin has been blamed for a lull in the development of surgical techniques in that period, as surgeons reached for the paraffin rather than the scalpel. However, over time the paraffin could reshape into localised lumps, or patients could experience inflammation and swelling.

The main attraction of injectables, which has remained unchanged, was the speed of the result. But over time the products used in these early attempts were found to be prone to complications, some of them serious. Injectables were discarded until safer and more effective products led to their huge resurgence in the late twentieth century—a resurgence that shows no signs of abating.

Fat injecting, or lipoinfiltration, has been in use for over fifteen years, but its use has recently taken on a new dimension with the unexpected discovery that fat contains stem cells and a large number of healing growth factors. Research is underway to learn how to capitalise on the enormous potential offered by fat and appears to be heading in the direction of tissue regeneration.

Our understanding of facial ageing is still progressing, but it's fair to say that much has been achieved over the past few decades to bring about a natural rejuvenation even on areas previously considered resistant to surgery, such as the neck. Our techniques to effect rejuvenation change constantly and each discovery by a surgeon opens a new window to our understanding, but in the end we need to consider just how far we really want to go in rejuvenation. The reality is, despite some exaggerated looks in the media, most patients just want to look ten years younger while retaining their natural looks and appearing simply to have aged well for their years.

16

A split in the specialty

Progress imposes not only new possibilities
for the future but new restrictions.

Norbert Wiener

A belief that aesthetic plastic surgery caters to an extreme form of vanity has deterred some surgeons from specialising in the field. Many have seen it as a service that panders to people who are not sick and are therefore unworthy of surgery. Surgeons who do provide aesthetic services have risked being dismissed as practising on the income-hungry periphery of 'real' surgery and viewed as outsiders rather than part of the mainstream, little more than expensive beauticians.

There is no doubt, of course, that the publicity-seeking behaviour of some of the early practitioners made it hard for the establishment to relate to them. Becoming an aesthetic plastic surgeon was something like going over to the dark side. For many years, eminent plastic surgeons who dealt daily with cancers and traumas in large teaching hospitals would disappear for an afternoon each week to rather furtively perform a few hours of aesthetic plastic surgery, away from their normal environment. They did so because they enjoyed the surgery or the financial profit—or both—but they didn't want to be seen doing it. As US plastic surgeon Robert Goldwyn noted, 'aesthetic surgery historically became like masturbation, practiced but not acknowledged'.

In 1958, Benjamin Rank (later Sir Benjamin), doyen among Australian plastic surgeons, wrote in the *Medical Journal of Australia* that

> facelifting has little, if any place in the surgical repertoire ... Looked at in perspective it is a procedure which would be better stamped out of common talk and thinking altogether.

His words reflected the fairly common view that aesthetic surgery was plastic surgery 'lite'. In the mid-1970s Rank prominently walked out of a presentation on breast implant surgery at the Annual Plastic Surgery Conference in Australia, cogently demonstrating his dismissive attitude towards the field. In those days, a woman could, after a mastectomy, feel traumatised and depressed by the sight of her ugly, scarred chest, but the medical world's common attitude was that saving the woman's life was enough. Her distress was seen as ingratitude, when in truth she was trying to rebuild her life as a normal social person, not just a medical survivor. Plastic surgery, by restoring her body in an aesthetic and emotional sense, could complete the process begun by her life-saving surgery.

Of course, times have changed and there has been increasing emphasis on quality of life as it affects the individual. Much of modern surgery falls into this category, such as the developments in orthopaedic surgery that are not immediately life saving but relieve pain and increase mobility so patients can participate fully in life.

Face-saving surgeon

One country that stands out as an exception to the reconstructive– aesthetic plastic surgery divide is Brazil, where there is a clear and widespread understanding of the link between facial appearance and overall health and happiness. Brazilians on the whole see aesthetic plastic surgery as being an integral part of plastic surgery and therefore deserving the same respect, due largely to a national tragedy that occurred in 1961.

In December of that year, in Niterói, Rio de Janeiro, a fire broke out inside a circus tent in which hundreds of children were gathered to watch a performance. Over three hundred people died and more than five hundred were injured. In the aftermath, local plastic surgeon Ivo Pitanguy emerged as a national hero as he worked to save the appearances of the children disfigured by burns. Pitanguy famously observed that a plastic surgeon is really a psychologist with a scalpel in his hands, and he demonstrated, through his work with the children, the ability of aesthetic plastic surgery to bring health to a suffering psyche. This bolstered widespread cultural acceptance in Brazil that human health means not merely physical health but also mental and sexual health, and even 'aesthetic health'. Since that time, living out his belief that the poor have a right to be beautiful, Pitanguy has run a clinic providing discounted aesthetic treatment to those who can't otherwise afford it. The Brazilian government also provides access to free cosmetic treatments in public hospitals.

There is no other living plastic surgeon so revered worldwide as Ivo Pitanguy. He trained in the United Kingdom, mainland Europe and the United States, and with his charm, confident manner and exceptional skills established a clinic in Rio in the 1960s that has drawn clientele from all around the world, including Hollywood, and which is the envy of other surgeons. Brazil has the largest number of plastic surgeons per head of population in the world. Pitanguy has trained more plastic surgeons than anyone else, and, importantly, through his influence, the Brazilian Society of Plastic Surgeons embraced the idea of aesthetic plastic surgery at the outset.

Further deepening of the divide between the worlds of reconstructive and aesthetic plastic surgery came about in the 1970s because of the changes occurring within aesthetic surgery itself. As we have seen, new solutions to the problems of the surgery were emerging. Its practitioners were no longer performing simple surgery on the skin; indeed, their research was beginning to change our entire understanding of the anatomy of the human face. The traditional notion of the general plastic surgeon was also starting to fragment due to rapid growth at the fringes of the specialty, with the emergence of the new subspecialties of craniofacial surgery and microsurgery. These specialties also involved a new anatomical understanding and attracted the brightest young plastic surgeons in the large university-based teaching hospitals where the procedures were performed. Tord Skoog's advances also gave face lifts greater respectability among plastic surgeons as the procedure took on a new dimension, becoming more complex and challenging. In order to perform a Skoog face lift, surgeons needed to have excellent anatomical knowledge as well as surgical skills.

No longer could the plastic surgeons who performed aesthetic surgery to this level be cast as mere 'wrinkle stretchers'.

Until that point, positions in the teaching hospitals, as well as the key leadership positions in the plastic surgery societies and conferences, were controlled by the 'establishment group', whose focus was on reconstructive plastic surgery. But in order to share their expanding knowledge and ideas, aesthetic surgeons needed specialist professional societies and journals. Without access to conferences, it is almost impossible for surgeons to teach and learn new techniques. Those on the aesthetic side of the divide struggled to have their ideas published or presented in more generalised forums; without access to publication they were unable to share their research, create teaching groups or disseminate ideas.

A permanent division in the world of plastic surgery was inevitable. By the end of the 1970s, nearly every Western country ended up with two or more plastic surgery societies: the traditional 'main' society, a society for aesthetic plastic surgery, and often a society for microsurgeons. The American Society for Aesthetic Plastic Surgery was founded in 1972, the International Society of Aesthetic Plastic Surgery in 1976 and the Australian Society of Aesthetic Plastic Surgery in 1977. Ironically, changing times and the growing number of plastic surgeons who specialise in aesthetic surgery have led to the mainstream societies now openly encouraging aesthetic surgery, so the basis for the original division no longer exists; there have even been moves to reunite. But the split in the late 1970s marked the beginning of an important new phase for aesthetic plastic surgery, demonstrating that it had effectively come of age almost a century after it started its journey with the work of such great individuals as John Orlando Roe and Jacques Joseph.

Part 3

Aesthetic plastic surgery today

Every face promises revelation.

Vivien Gaston

17

Patients

Presume not that I am the thing I was.

William Shakespeare

R eliable statistics are hard to come by, but it seems likely that between 80 and 90 per cent of aesthetic surgery patients are female, and that most of those having facial surgery (rather than non-surgical procedures such as injectables) are between thirty-five and sixty years old. Rhinoplasty patients tend to be younger, however: between their late teens and early thirties.

According to the International Society of Aesthetic Plastic Surgery, in 2010 blepharoplasty (eyelid surgery) and rhino-plasty were the most commonly performed facial plastic surgery procedures in the world. When grouped with all surgi-cal procedures carried out by plastic surgeons—including all parts of the body and not just the face—in Brazil, China, India and Japan both blepharoplasty and rhinoplasty were among the top five most common procedures. Worldwide, blepharoplasty was the third most popular procedure (behind liposuction and breast augmentation) of all aesthetic procedures, accounting for 11 per cent of all surgical procedures, and rhinoplasty was the fourth most popular, making up 10 per cent of all procedures. Abdominoplasty (tummy tuck) finished off the top five, with the face lift being the next facial procedure on the list, in eighth place, accounting for 4 per cent of all surgical procedures.

Similar but not identical results were found in the United States in 2011 by the American Society for Aesthetic Plastic Surgery. It also found that the facial surgical procedure most frequently performed by plastic surgeons was blepharoplasty. However, this was the only facial surgery to appear in the top five of all plastic surgery procedures, behind liposuction, breast augmentation and abdominoplasty, and ahead of breast reduction. Rhinoplasty was sixth on the list, with the face lift seventh and the brow or forehead lift tenth. Within the top five surgeries for men in the United States were two facial procedures: rhinoplasty and blepharoplasty, while women had only one facial procedure in the top five, which was blepharoplasty.

Non-surgical procedures dominated the picture of facial procedures in the United States in 2011, with 2.5 million procedures using botulinum toxin type A (botox) against 150,000 blepharoplasties. In reality that's probably only a fraction of the true figure for non-surgical procedures, for it may not take into account injecting performed by assistants and specialist nurses within plastic surgery clinics, as well as myriad other non-specialist places that offer injecting in the community. Non-surgical procedures had grown rapidly, contributing to media reports about the rise in cosmetic procedures in general. In the United States, between 1997 and 2011, while surgical procedures rose by 73 per cent, non-surgical procedures increased by 356 per cent.

One of the problems with data about facial surgery is that it is performed by many different sorts of surgeons—and even doctors without a surgical qualification—so statistics from plastic surgeons may only reflect a part of the true picture. Ear, nose and throat surgeons, for instance, perform many rhinoplasties and some perform the full range of facial procedures. Some dermatologists also perform procedures that can be aesthetic in nature. In addition, there are the 'cosmetic surgeons' who don't have a surgical degree but still have practices dedicated entirely to aesthetic surgery.

Patient profiles

Despite the mass media telling a different story, aesthetic plastic surgery patients are not all actors and celebrities, or the vain and entitled. Instead, they are people from all sections of the community who have surgery for all sorts of reasons. They are rarely wealthy, and their surgery is a significant expenditure that has to be considered carefully. Often, they have had to overcome a personal distaste for the very idea of plastic surgery. But they have reached a point in their lives where their appearance is holding them back in some way, or affecting their ability to fully enjoy their lives. This can be due to having lived through a devastating event or it can arise internally, from a simple desire to look better than they do. The need to improve or perfect facial appearance is, after all, a universal aspect of human nature. All societies and cultures express this, even in its simplest form as decoration of the face. It's the reason people wear makeup—to highlight their best features in order to appear more attractive

than they might naturally be. Extensive research on the subject
by sociologist Beverley McNamara concluded that 'all people
seek, to some degree, to decorate and change the body shape,
size and surface and that this continues through time'. It's not
such a major step to think of aesthetic surgery as a continuation
of this—people meeting a need inside themselves for aesthetic
satisfaction.

Plastic surgery has been best described as surgery of the
emotions—in fact, psychosurgery. Patients seek a surgical solution to a physical problem that manifests in emotional ways.
Unlike most surgical patients, they're usually physically healthy,
but something in their physical appearance is negatively affecting the very centre of their lives and social functioning.

Living live to the full

Patient consultations can have their humorous moments, particularly,
I've found, with more elderly women. Many of these, I often discover
after surgery, are older than they told me initially, but they prudently
fudge their age to ensure I agree to their operations. They're great characters, enjoying life to the full and proof of the new attitude to ageing that
is causing much of the growth in plastic surgery. One woman confessed
after her face lift that she had lied about her age and was not eighty-
four; she was actually eighty-eight. 'My father said that a woman should
always lie about her age,' she said, before telling me about her (much
younger) lover and her desire to have a bit of a 'touch-up' procedure in
what she referred to as her 'privates'. Then she laughed. 'Well, actually,'
she said, 'they're not all *that* private'.

For many patients, the road to the plastic surgeon's door
involves a complex and emotional journey, initially—and

perhaps surprisingly—unrelated to a desire to change their facial appearance. Divorce, a major illness, the death of a parent (especially if they were that parent's carer) and even, as we will see, the death of a child—all such events, once the immediate trauma is over, remind people of the importance of life and the need to live it to the full. When they decide to move on, removing physical traces of stress or grief can be a pragmatic act to support their psychological and emotional wellbeing. They believe, and the available research supports this, that feeling better about their looks will help their confidence and self-esteem as they move into the future.

A surprising number of patients are mothers who have lost children. Their presence in the operating theatres of plastic surgeons defies the media-led ideas of the 'typical' plastic surgery patient. I personally see two or three every year. Sometimes bereaved mothers have surgery years after their loss, by which time their suffering is visibly etched on their faces. I can usually see it as soon as they walk into the consulting room. It raises the question: can plastic surgery really help someone who has suffered the death of a child? The role, and benefit, of aesthetic plastic surgery in instances like this is that it can help to smooth out one area of life and, by doing so, play a beneficial role in that person's subsequent fate. For the patients who have lived through difficulties such as this, the timing of their surgery can be important. Frequently, help from a psychiatrist or psychologist is necessary to ensure they have recovered sufficiently from the trauma they have faced and are ready to take a significant step forwards, like surgery. Some, for instance after a divorce, feel a certain urgency, a result of the 'wasted' years behind them, and want to move on as quickly as possible; others, such as those who have experienced a family death, move more slowly.

Telltale eyes of grief

My nineteen-month-old son died when I was twenty-seven. It was so sudden and devastating. I couldn't measure the profound grief that I felt. Six years later, to the very day, my mother died, after much suffering. And then, two years after that, my closest and dearest brother—we were like twins—was killed in an accident. All that grief. All that crying. Years of it. I struggled to get through the grief.

How can I separate my life experience from my decision to have surgery? It's not possible. The pain showed on my face. When I cried I could hardly see—I developed big 'eye bags' with just slits for eyes. I cried so much, my bags got bigger and my eyes got smaller. They became 'telltale eyes', expert at letting family, friends and the neighbourhood know how I was going.

I was judged all the time because of what had happened to me. People would say, 'Oh, you're the one whose child died'. There was no rest from it. They stopped seeing me and just saw the grief person. I know people are caring but it wears you out. I wore a lot of makeup so no-one could see how I was hurting, and my mask got thicker and thicker—I used to talk about putting on my mask before going out—and I never wanted to take my glasses off. I thought I looked awful, like my whole life was written on my face.

I kept on going, as a wife, mum and employee and for a while forgot how I looked. But my eyes—which were always deep set— now felt heavy, slitty, clogged up as if they were full of fluid, with puffy lids and huge bags underneath. While they looked like that, the comments kept coming, reminding me that my pain was right there on my face.

Initially I wanted the surgery to improve my vision, let the light in more ... but also I wanted to feel better. After surgery the grief was still there, of course—but now I feel as if I'm in control of the grief rather than it being right there in everyone's face. I feel that because I look better I can control it better.

Patients who seek aesthetic surgery solely because they are disatissfied with their face often come in knowing exactly what they want and express it easily: 'I hate my nose', 'I'm sick of people telling me I look tired', or 'I hate the bags under my eyes'. Their answer to the question 'Why now?' may be as simple as having finally found the time, money or confidence to get it done. Such patients approach surgery from an aesthetic perspective, requesting specific improvements to make their face more attractive or better aligned with the person they perceive themselves to be. These people tend to have a good aesthetic eye and an appreciation of detail, so their judgement is usually correct: there *is* some aspect of their face that looks out of place or just plain wrong, spoiling its overall proportions. Their decision to have it corrected is positive, and surgery is a self-improvement that allows them to get on with life with more confidence.

Culture and geography also play a role in what people want from their surgery. In some areas of the United States, such as Los Angeles, Miami and Dallas, the exaggerated and overly perfect look of glamour that we see on some Hollywood actors and celebrities is actively sought, but the same look would be shunned in conservative areas such as Boston. In Brazil, the 'tight' look is prized. In general, however, I meet people who want a subtle result that is natural-looking and imperceptible to others. Of course, this may reflect only my own practice's end of the surgical spectrum, as surgeons do become known for their style, but nine out of ten of my patients say they want to look like themselves, but attractively so.

There are some people for whom aesthetic surgery—whatever the procedure and whenever they may seek it—is simply the wrong option. As we saw earlier, estimates suggest that up to 15 per cent of people seeking aesthetic plastic surgery suffer from body dysmorphic disorder. They do not gain the satisfaction usually associated with aesthetic surgery, and for that reason should not be operated upon. But they are not the only people who are not good candidates for surgery. Some people suffer from unresolved angers or anxieties, or emotional conditions that require appropriate help before surgery can be of assistance. As the plastic surgeon Robert M Goldwyn remarked, 'for some patients surgery can be a metaphor for something else, and the doctor can unwittingly participate in the wrong scenario'. This is very true and plastic surgeons are becoming increasingly alert to the need to ensure patients are psychologically ready for surgery and that surgery itself is the correct course of action. It isn't possible to operate successfully on a delusion.

Recovery

Whatever procedure patients undergo, they want to recover in peace and quiet and then slip unnoticed back into their lives. Fear of being ridiculed or caught out is naturally high, and most patients feel some degree of embarrassment about having plastic surgery. Many want a 'quick fix' and a rapid recovery, and usually hope to squeeze the surgery into a two-week hiatus in their commitments. Since Charles Willi's triumphant 'half an hour for half a new face', the approach of most surgeons has been to make the operations faster, less inconvenient and less expensive; generally, to have them fit in with the instant gratification world we live in. But surgeons do vary in the degree of compromise they will accept. A quick recovery necessitates minimal surgery, but this can lead to patient unhappiness if the result fails to live up to their hopes.

Unfortunately, nature sets the pace for recovery, however quick the patient might will it to be. It can be a testing time for patients, when many undergo not just physical discomfort but emotional ups and downs that can be quite significant. It is not possible to change something that is so inextricably a part of individual identity without undergoing some level of psychological disturbance. Patients need support from their surgeon and, where possible, from family or a friend. Surgery is, of necessity, a step into the unknown. The patient trades one situation for another, in the hope that it's beneficial for them. Until the benefit is realised, and the patient can see that the decision was a good one, the situation is understandably stressful.

For the surgeon, the best day is day five after a patient's surgery. Swelling builds up for the first three post-operative days but has perceptibly eased when the patient wakes up on the fifth day. Not only does the face feel less tight, but the patient feels better, as if getting over the flu, and they experience the first sense of optimism about the outcome. At day five, they find confidence to believe that everything is working as they'd hoped.

Procedures

The aesthetic plastic surgeon, by agreeing to operate, takes on some of the responsibility for their patient's decision. They can contribute positively to a patient's future, or make it worse. Either way, they are implicated in the process: in a sense, their name is on their patient's face.

Sometimes during the consultation process, patients express dissatisfaction with one part of their face when in fact the surgeon knows that they would benefit more from surgical attention to a different part. Practical procedure-related issues such as this can present the surgeon with a real dilemma. Should they, based on their years of experience, mention those other areas of potential correction that would be beneficial to the patient's appearance? It's not the surgeon's role to make the patient feel uncomfortable or to end up inadvertently discouraging them from having any surgery at all: patients come to see a surgeon for help, and if they're turned off the idea of surgery they haven't been helped at all and are denied the benefit that surgery might have given them.

An area in which this dilemma frequently crops up is with jowls, known as 'jawls' in old English—the sagging laxity of skin over the jawline. Women whose mothers or grandmothers had this problem often dread the arrival of jowls on their own face, almost waiting for the first signs, at which stage they may perceive worse deterioration than actually exists. It's often the case that such patients would benefit more overall from having a blepharoplasty than from having the jowls removed, but the latter attends to their emotional needs as much as to their true surgical needs. The surgeon's limits and role in such cases are not always clear, and they sometimes wonder whether patients will mostly feel relieved that they've fixed their jowls, or disappointed that they don't look quite as rejuvenated as they'd hoped.

This leads us to an interesting point about the intersection of procedures. Sometimes, at first glance, procedures suggested by plastic surgeons to correct an abnormality or improve a feature may appear to have no relationship to each other. Combining a blepharoplasty and a brow lift is one such example. The upper eyelid's appearance is influenced both by the lid itself and by the position of the brow above it, so if a patient wants to improve the appearance of their eyelids the surgeon needs to decide what proportion of the appearance is due to the lids and what proportion to the brow. If the lids are responsible for, say, 80 per cent of the unsatisfactory appearance and the brow 20 per cent, if the patient opts for only a blepharoplasty they can expect up to an 80 per cent improvement. Difficulties can arise when the problem stems equally from the brow and the lids: for a satisfactory result, the surgeon is almost obliged to correct both. But for the patient, the situation has suddenly changed. Having thought they would just need a blepharoplasty, they're now looking at a more complex—and more costly—operation if they want guaranteed improvement.

Patient satisfaction

The first studies of plastic surgery results appeared in 1940, and these were followed by further research over the next two decades. They were based on psychiatrist interviews and found that most patients had significant psychopathology, including depression, anxiety and low self-esteem, before surgery. After surgery, the symptoms of these conditions increased. It seemed a poor start to the boom years of plastic surgery. It turned out, however, that a flawed methodology had been used, which frequently displayed bias by the interviewers and led to premature conclusions about the patients' mental state. As a result, the studies have now been largely discounted, but it's possible that their shadow lingers: there is ongoing reluctance to believe that people can be happier as a result of plastic surgery.

Meaningful data is still hard to find, reflecting the complexity of the research that would be needed. Studies in the 1970s found that women benefit, with less depression and anxiety post-operatively. A study by the American Society for Aesthetic Plastic Surgery published in 2006 claimed that women who had aesthetic surgery such as rhinoplasty or face lift and including breast augmentation and body contouring experienced a high degree of body image satisfaction after surgery. For those undergoing the surgery, there was an added bonus of greater sexual satisfaction, but sadly this was less noticeable for those who had undergone facial surgery.

Attempts are being made to develop a statistically valid means of measuring face lift patient satisfaction. As a step towards this, a study was undertaken in 2010 to follow up SMAS face lift patients who had undergone surgery between January 1994 and January 1999. Almost 98 per cent of the patients contacted reported satisfaction levels of 'very good' or 'beyond expectations' after one year, and nearly 70 per cent at twelve years. Younger patients consistently gave more positive ratings and reported greater overall satisfaction, despite the fact that they were found to be the most reluctant in the first place to undertake the surgery required.

Reactions

Research carried out in 2011 by the American Society for Aesthetic Plastic Surgery reported that 51 per cent of Americans said they approved of cosmetic plastic surgery, and 67 per cent said they would not be embarrassed if their friends knew they'd had it performed. However, few people in society are without an opinion on aesthetic facial surgery, and when a person decides to have it, their choice can arouse strong emotions in family and friends, who can be a source of great support or another struggle the patient has to overcome. Suzanne Noël, the plastic surgeon who was based in Paris in the early twentieth century, made the interesting observation that American and British husbands were happy to send their wives to have surgery, but French husbands bristled with resistance against it.

Facial surgery can illuminate the hierarchy within patients' lives, or upset the pecking order of their group, either because of the improved appearance of the person or simply because the decision itself revealed something about their personality that hadn't been previously known. This occurred in the bridge group of one of my patients: she was the oldest in the group, but after surgery she no longer looked the oldest, and this led to a considerable amount of feather ruffling among the younger members. The firm but unacknowledged order around the bridge table had been shaken by her action.

Some of it naturally comes back to the observations made by the plastic surgeon Maxwell Maltz that surgery could assist but not ensure change; the key was whether the patient's self-image had changed along with the surgery. Nearly thirty years before he wrote the self-help bestseller *Psycho-Cybernetics* he wrote about patients and their experience of post-surgical satisfaction in *New Faces, New Futures: Rebuilding character with plastic surgery* (1936).

Surgery, no matter how good, obviously can't substitute for a life poorly lived or values that simply don't lead to happiness. But, in general, I have found that if people have a specific problem from which they want relief, and if their expectations are aligned with surgical reality, the chances are high that they will feel happier as a result. One day, as I was leaving the office, a woman tapped on my car window. 'I know you probably don't remember me,' she said, 'but you did my face lift sixteen years ago and I have thanked you every day since, when I look in the mirror'. Such comments, apart from greatly motivating the surgeon, show that sometimes people just need a bit of help at a certain time of their life. It doesn't make them victims of an appearance-obsessed culture, but identifies them as people who have made and benefited from a practical decision.

18

Surgeons

The plastic surgeon is undoubtedly the
greatest of all contemporary artists.
He paints on living canvas and sculpts in
human flesh contributing to the health and
happiness and success of his patient.

Charles Willi

The International Society of Aesthetic Plastic Surgery estimated that in 2010 there were 33,000 plastic surgeons worldwide. The country with the largest proportion of these—18 per cent—was the United States, which was closely followed by Brazil, then India, China and Japan. Australia ranked twenty-second, with just over two hundred plastic surgeons, slightly ahead of Saudi Arabia, the Netherlands and Romania. According to the society's figures, Australian plastic surgeons performed over 61,000 surgical procedures in 2010.

Requirements

A plastic surgeon needs an artistic eye, imagination, creativity and a sense of aesthetics, claimed the renowned Brazilian surgeon Ivo Pitanguy. In the end, the aesthetic plastic surgeon who does not appreciate beauty is probably working in the wrong field. We are not the arbiters of beauty, but its spirit guides us and if we can restore attractiveness to someone's face, then we feel delight for them and satisfaction for what we do.

Another important characteristic in a plastic surgeon is expressed in my personal motto: *dedication to the total eradication of all errors*. Infinite care over every aspect of their treatment is what patients expect and are entitled to receive. But the rewards for surgeons are also great. Each time I perform facial surgery I feel like an explorer, excited to be the first person in there, deep in the tissues of the face; the anatomy itself is beautiful, and every face, although possessed of the same anatomy, is slightly different. I may have done a procedure innumerable times, but it never loses its thrill—a good procedure, provided it is done well, is inherently satisfying to a plastic surgeon. Recognition for our work tends to come from our patients, whose gratitude is expressed behind closed doors. Their words are frequent reminders of the importance of what we do, and reflect the unique position aesthetic surgery occupies at the crossroads between surgery and psychology, addressing the person as well as their appearance.

This is not something surgery has traditionally excelled at. In fact, in a busy hospital, a patient could sometimes more aptly be described as the vehicle for a surgical problem, and they may scarcely meet the surgeon beforehand. If the surgeon is proficient and removes their diseased gall bladder quickly and efficiently, it's probably enough. But aesthetic plastic surgery is quite different. Not only is the time that the surgeon spends with the patient critical to their happiness, but the quality of the surgery needs to be exceptionally high to achieve the desired result. If you can see what has been done, the surgeon has failed. Some of the finest craft work in surgery is performed by plastic surgeons, in microsurgery, cleft lip surgery and aesthetic facial surgery especially. It requires a technical proficiency and a degree of meticulous attention to detail that are less critical in some other areas of surgery. Of course, getting it right is always the prime aim of any surgeon, but getting it right and invisible on the most visible part of the body is another matter altogether. The two great plastic surgeons Harold Gillies and D Ralph Millard Jr wrote about the intrinsic need for perfection in aesthetic surgery and reminded us that

> It is easier to reduce than to produce, but in plastic surgery it is nearly always necessary to remould after reduction. Thus anyone can cut off a bit of a nose or breast, but not so many can turn out a satisfying result.

Plastic surgeons find themselves in an inherently stressful situation. The result of surgery has to look excellent, and the patient has to be pleased, *because their future happiness is at stake*. It's a potent situation. Much of the surgeon's time is spent working with patients who are anxious and prone to moments of great uncertainty, having made a decision that will affect their looks and their future. The unusual situation of the face, as an emotional as well as a physical space, forms the critical backdrop to the surgeon's everyday working environment.

Surgical damage

I was a fifty-three-year-old receptionist who loved working and was in the public eye: I was single, very happy and contented with my life. After discussing the idea with friends and reading a little on the subject, I decided that I wanted to freshen up my appearance, to achieve a more even skin tone without makeup, and remove puffiness from above and below my eyes. After consulting two plastic surgeons I underwent simultaneous eye surgery and facial lasering. After the inevitable swelling and bruising of the procedures subsided, it became increasingly apparent that there was damage arising from the procedures.

The shock I felt as the disfigurement of the surgery became apparent was devastating. My self-confidence plummeted and my distress continued to increase as the doctors and physicians I approached for help advised either that there was nothing that could be done, or that they were unwilling to try or to become involved in my case.

After negotiations one of these surgeons performed a further two operations to rectify the original mistakes. But during these procedures nerves in my face were damaged, causing the right side to be partially paralysed and the brow and eye on that side to droop. There was also loss of movement in my top and bottom lips and on the right side of my neck. My whole appearance was now quite lopsided.

After three years of this I had gone from being confident, outgoing and happy to only being able to hold myself together while at work. When I saw my face, there was always, for me, the daily and starkly visible reminder of the surgery and the professional disregard I had experienced. I became despondent and depressed, increasingly isolated and desperate. I lost over four years of my life and ended up tens of thousands of dollars out of pocket.

[After further successful surgery,] where the right side of my face had previously been somewhat immobile and droopy, there was immediately a noticeable, positive difference to the symmetry of

my face. I felt as if I had a new lease on life, reinvigorated and more confident, with less sense that people were looking at my odd facial appearance. Finally, I was able to look into the mirror and see my face emerging without focusing on the disfigurements. There was an immense sense of relief that I now appeared normal, even glamorous and attractive, which gave me much personal satisfaction. And as my face emerged so did I, with increasing confidence and a feeling of self-worth that I had not felt for a very long time. I felt I was coming out of the shadows of an abyss and into the full light of a normal day. I dare not think where I might be today if I had not had that corrective surgery.

The surgeon–patient relationship

The surgeon–patient relationship is at the centre of the aesthetic plastic surgery experience. Without doubt, the manner in which the service is delivered is as important as the objective result. Technical success and a great result will not make a patient happy unless their perception of the process was also positive. This reflects the profound psychological dimensions of the choice to have facial surgery.

This relationship is essential to a successful outcome and starts in the first moments of the consultation. What patients divulge during a consultation is often highly personal, a real glimpse into the hidden dimensions of their life. In fact, that's the purpose of the consultation. Surgeons need to know what the person's motivation is and why they have chosen now to seek help. During one consultation, a woman suddenly told me that her son had been killed in an accident. 'I died for ten years,' she told me, unforgettably. This is what a consultation is about. The impact of that woman's words could not have been conveyed on a written form; nor would the information have surfaced at all if we had limited our discussion to the surgery. Information such as this is important because it creates an informed partnership between the surgeon and the patient. It's a lengthy partnership, as the surgeon becomes the patient's guide in all respects, from making the decision to the final return to normal life after surgery. In that time we get to know each other well, and at an intensity that could almost equal some marriages, as many patients experience moments of emotional fragility that they have never encountered before. This is most likely to occur in the early part of the healing phase, making plastic surgery one of the few surgical specialities requiring careful after-care of the emotions, tending to the psyche and not just the surgical outcome. This extends to every staff member, as everyone encountered in association with the surgery is seen to be an extension of the surgical process. The patient's perception of the process is only as strong as their weakest experience during it, and any awareness of an interruption in good communication may upset their confidence in the whole.

Legal issues

Surgery is not like landing a plane, or a mechanical situation where if you do the same thing each time you get the same result. Surgery is a complex procedure in which the patient's own body, healing and post-operative activities play their part in the recovery process and, therefore, the final outcome. The result is not always what either the surgeon or the patient intended. For the surgeon, this has the potential to end a career.

A top aesthetic plastic surgeon in Dallas who specialised in taking on the most difficult problems, either fixing up previous surgery performed by other surgeons or taking patients referred to him because of the surgical challenges involved, experienced the devastation that can be wrought by an unhappy patient. The surgeon's results were consistently outstanding, and he taught a generation of plastic surgeons, but there's a limit to what can be achieved in very complex cases; the most-sued practitioners in neurosurgery and other higher risk specialities are not those taking the general cases but those working on the major, complicated cases. A highly aggrieved patient, who was actually in part responsible for an unsatisfactory healing on his nose, set up a website highly critical of the surgeon, and it was the first site listed every time a potential patient googled the surgeon's name. The surgeon continued to work, but the public perception of his abilities gained from a Google search was very different to the reality and some potential patients were no doubt dissuaded and lost the benefit of his work.

In Australia, since the early 1990s, the legal situation has been clear: surgeons are required to explain all the relevant considerations—namely, the risks—involved in their surgery, so that patients are fully aware of every possible outcome as they go about deciding whether to have an operation. The law came about through a renowned Australian legal case, *Rogers v Whitaker* (1992), which changed the legal dynamic of the patient–surgeon consultation. In this tragic case, a woman who originally had vision only in her left eye underwent surgery to try to improve the vision in, and the appearance of, her right eye. Although the surgery was conducted with the required skill and care, the patient developed a rare condition leading to the loss of vision in both eyes.

In the ensuing legal case, the surgeon relied upon the principle that medical practitioners are not negligent if they act in accordance with practice accepted by their peers as being 'proper'. But the High Court of Australia ruled that all surgery (other than obvious exceptions such as emergency surgery) is preceded by a choice made by the patient. If the patient hasn't been given all the relevant information and advice, their choice is rendered meaningless. The court found that 'the Law should recognise that a medical practitioner has a duty to warn a patient of a material risk inherent in the proposed treatment', meaning that even a very remote risk normally dismissed by the surgeon as extremely unlikely to occur could be considered material to the patient who needs to decide whether to have surgery or not, and that it is the duty of the surgeon to disclose it.

This ruling was obviously a good decision but has ended up being difficult to uphold from a logistical and sometimes a practical point of view. Firstly, patients find themselves loaded with all sorts of information that is irrelevant to their specific concern. This level of information probably provides less comfort to patients than it does to the surgeon's insurer, whose requirements it fulfils. The law also presents the surgeon with a dilemma if they feel, during surgery, that deviating slightly from the surgery plan or adding a small extra procedure would benefit the patient: if it hasn't been explicitly discussed beforehand, the surgeon is now taking a large risk if they continue.

In every practice there are unhappy patients. Often they are the people you have most difficulty relating to and perhaps therein lies the problem, again one of psychology rather than surgery. A solution is usually found when the patient is given the opportunity to discuss how they feel and the surgeon listens carefully with the intent of helping rather than defending.

19

Plastic world

A plastic surgeon does not simply alter a man's face.
He alters the man's inner self. The incisions he makes
are more than skin deep. They frequently cut deep
into the psyche as well.

Maxwell Maltz

The growing presence of aesthetic surgery raises many questions in today's society; the media is almost obsessed with examples of its unwise or inappropriate use, and some social commentators are concerned by the values they believe underlie it. Their viewpoints are well summarised by Anthony Elliott, professor of sociology at Flinders University, South Australia, in his book *Making the Cut: How cosmetic surgery is transforming our lives*. Their central concern is that plastic surgery builds and intensifies a restless culture built on superficial anxieties about appearance—a culture that reveres ceaseless renovation over hard work, experience and a secure sense of individual identity. In short, it's a fear that we could be heading for a 'soulless surgical world' lacking in contemplation and depth, and based on the desire for (and delivery of) immediate results. Some of the more driven aspects of American society are used as examples, such as the constant demand for self-improvement, which leads to a competitive 'treadmill' society, in which exhausted members struggle to keep up. That much-heard retort, 'that is so yesterday!' says it all. Yesterday and everything you learnt yesterday are just not important.

This places plastic surgery deep within the culture of globalisation, in which old certainties, such as a job for life, loyalty to the individual and reward for effort, have no place. In this world, older people naturally feel devalued and increasingly anxious about their position, so they may believe there is no option but to conceal their true age. Male plastic surgery patients are cited as an example of people under this pressure, choosing surgery to secure their work prospects as they age. But, as we've seen, there's nothing new in this. Workplace security was one of the earliest motivations for rejuvenation surgery in both men and women, as Suzanne Noël wrote. The other way of looking at it is that surgery can actually help people of any age to secure their future—if their face is holding them back in some way. I was recently visited by a man I had operated on twenty-two years earlier. During those years he had completed a PhD at a top American university and gone on to an exceptional career in his chosen field. He told me that he believed his surgery as a young man was the single most important decision leading to that success. It was a classic instance of the right surgery at the right time helping a person along their path in life.

Beauty in Brazil

It is claimed that plastic surgery has changed society in Brazil. There, beauty has become a 'democratiser', giving people at the bottom of a stratified social structure the opportunity to rise in ways never before possible. Whereas class and race previously determined one's future, now beauty and style have social value, and someone with no other means to rise can use plastic surgery to enhance their chances. It's a form of currency—pulchronomics on a social scale—changing the power structures in society. Despite this 'beauty mobility', the spread of surgery through the general population creates some discomfort, with the wealthier (who also embrace plastic surgery) considering it vulgar in others. But it's an irresistible force. Television shows and celebrity culture displaying poor people made good ensure that this thinking remains part of modern experience, even in very poor countries. This crossover between plastic surgery, celebrity culture and notions of the good life can seem indicative of an empty existence to those of us from more affluent societies, but in socially stratified societies that place a premium on the physical body, its economic and social enticement is more understandable.

The 'anti–plastic surgery' viewpoint is concerned that consumerism is recasting our true identity, so that it's now actually created by (and catered to by) cosmetics, clothing, therapists, gyms and surgeons. While industries such as cosmetics make billions of dollars out of this need to 'create' our identity, the end result is, of course, only more emptiness—we seek the next thing, then the next thing, without ever finding anything worthwhile. In its place is a new culture, a 'culture of inauthenticity', in which a celebrity's artificial breasts can bring her worldwide notice. As celebrities acquire fame and fortune through surgically created attributes, young and attractive people are suddenly no longer satisfied with their own looks but want to emulate something that never naturally existed in the first place.

It's normal to feel concerned about this sort of world. It has the values and priorities of an unhappy society that anyone in the modern Western world can recognise—a place in which good sense and proper ideals seem to have no place. As surgeon Robert Goldwyn acknowledged nearly thirty years ago, plastic surgery does have an ambivalent role in this trivialised, image-conscious world: both creating the demand and catering to it.

But it's a societal problem that needs to be met by society on a larger canvas than just plastic surgery. It's about deciding what sort of society we want, not what sort of surgery. To be human is to be in a state of constant change, so it's understandable that our society is also endlessly changing. Our new awareness of brain plasticity shows that our own brain is continuously changing, re-forming with each experience and memory. As novelist Richard Powers describes it in *The Echo Maker*, 'the brain that retrieved a memory was not the brain that had formed it. Even retrieving a memory mangled what was formerly there'. Maybe we are in a state of constant restlessness and the difference is that we now have the means to act upon it.

The potential for abuse occurs when people are not able to think for themselves or make sensible judgements about their own lives. In that instance, facial surgery may look like a fast track, to be used at whim by some people to meet poor-quality desires. Without ethical restraints, plastic surgery could become twisted into a short-term 'fix' in this unstable world, helping people to cope and feeding their anxiety at the same time. The array of ever-more affordable and available aesthetic treatments will force us to confront issues such as the ethical behaviour of the surgeons—or, increasingly, the non-specialists—who dispense them. But to overreact to this possibility would be to deny the people who we've discussed in this book, for whom aesthetic surgery has offered a way of living that is based on a genuine desire to live well as a good person.

Another aspect of the 'plastic world' is sameness—the idea that we could all end up looking the same, almost like plastic people. With proper surgery this doesn't happen, but the possibility exists, certainly in theory, if enough people deliberately choose one particular look. However, as only a minute percentage of the population actually undergoes aesthetic surgery, it remains in the realms of theory. People prize their individuality, and patients definitely fear losing their identity. But the overuse of a particular product or procedure can inadvertently lead to an amorphous look which we see in the excessive use of fillers or fat injections in older women, swelling their face until it looks bland and without the individuality they had in youth.

Surgical sameness

Some cities have pockets of 'surgical sameness', usually resulting from a dominant local surgeon whose training of other surgeons ends up disproportionately influencing the appearance of patients in that area, as their work spreads across the population.

The 'Dallas nose' is one example: an extremely refined, almost exaggerated nose tip. People with the nose retain their individual appearance but also look strangely the same. It's disconcerting, and unmistakable once you start to notice it. The nose came about through the work of Jack Gunter, a superb rhinoplasty surgeon, who operated and also taught many other surgeons in Dallas, Texas, creating a concentration of cases, even though his influence was worldwide.

A patient of mine once asked for a secondary rhinoplasty (surgery to improve a previous rhinoplasty) prompted by walking past a woman who had an identical nose to hers. She vividly described her dismay at realising that her 'new' nose was in fact just a signature of the surgeon who had created it. My task was to remove that surgeon's signature and replace it with a nose that suited her face.

The situation can also occur when patients seek a particular look. In New York City in the 1980s, women frequently had face lifts that included the upper eyelid surgery popular at the time. They were photographed for magazines like *Town and Country*, all featuring a distinctive haughty, imperial look. Their exaggeratedly deep-set eyes were not the result of any aristocratic gene pool, but the legacy of a sought-after facial rejuvenation that gave a predictably standard result.

Finally, there's the issue of fakery—the unease that many people feel about a copy or reworking compared to an original item. When a forgery is passed off as an original, the audience feels duped, or tricked. Plastic surgery raises the question of whether we are seeing the 'real' person, or just what they want us to see while they remain out of sight behind their enhanced exterior. Knowing the real age of a person still matters; it tells us something important about them and prepares our expectations. Many people hold to the notion that nature and age give us the face intended for us. In reality, plastic surgery can make an appearance difference of about ten years, so a middle-aged person still looks middle-aged, just a better-aged version. It's not a sleight of hand. Many recipients of plastic surgery would say that their face lift revealed the real them. If the post-surgical appearance of a person's face brings it into alignment with the inner feelings of the person and allows them to live with greater confidence, then the surgery has done its work, irrespective of others' judgements.

For most patients, good-quality plastic surgery is a comfort, either an aid to wellbeing or an alleviation of suffering. It's certainly possible that life's transience can create an anxious desire to keep 'doing things', but this is not obvious in plastic surgeons' offices yet. Plastic surgery is rarely used to emulate a celebrity or step into some illusory world of reputation and wealth. Good sense prevails.

Afterword

The face lift operation

It only remained to conquer old age.

Aldous Huxley

The start of an operation is a quiet, purpose-filled time when all members of our small team are busy preparing for their roles in the operating theatre. The environment in theatre is extremely important, and I find I don't operate as smoothly without relaxing music in the background. Usually, we have Beethoven piano music playing to set a tranquil atmosphere before the patient arrives in the theatre. When I reach a key part of the operation, I'll have the volume reduced or the music switched off altogether. Some of the major procedures take up to five hours or more, with prolonged segments of intense concentration, so it's not just a matter of enjoying the music—it's about creating an environment for calm, focused attention.

At the beginning, the anaesthetist is centre stage, and I stand aside so they can give the intense focus to their work that it requires. The induction of an anaesthetic for an anaesthetist is not unlike a pilot on take-off: if anything goes wrong it can happen quickly. Fortunately, with their modern training and experience, this is a rare occurrence. While the anaesthetist is at work, I'm doing the final planning for the surgery and mentally rehearsing the sequence and the important variations in what I'm about to do. But I stay alert to what the anaesthetist is doing. In particular, I keep an eye on the computer monitor to watch the patient's blood pressure. We don't want it to rise significantly when the endotracheal (breathing) tube is put in the patient's airway. This sometimes happens, as it's inherently irritating to have a tube placed in the throat, even when unconscious. If it takes longer than normal, due to the patient having a difficult airway, it can stimulate a rise in the blood pressure. Even though the pressure will later fall, the effect is not the same as if it had remained stable. Some anaesthetists are more adept at inserting the tube than others, and some give the patient a beta-blocker drug to prevent the pressure rising.

Keeping the blood pressure low and controlled is important for facial surgery, just as it is in neurosurgery. Part of the anaesthetist's job is to keep the pressure within the target range so the surgeon can operate with minimum bleeding. If the patient bleeds, precious time is wasted in controlling the bleeding vessels, which is undesirable. Even a tiny bit of oozing blood limits visibility in critical areas. In addition, bleeding at the time of surgery causes bruising in the tissues, which slows the postoperative recovery. In some procedures, such as eyelid surgery, we aim to completely avoid bruising and can achieve this in 90 per cent of cases.

So an anaesthetist working in aesthetic plastic surgery has different priorities from a colleague working in, say, orthopaedics, where the operating environment does not need to be as precise and their priorities are to make the patient ready as quickly as possible, so the surgeon can get on with their work. Most plastic surgeons work with just a select few anaesthetists who have developed exceptional skills in maintaining the ideal plastic surgical environment.

Still keeping my eye on the blood pressure monitor, I place the sheet containing the surgical plan and a series of enlarged photos of the patient's face, taken from several angles, on a docket rail on the wall. They're there so I can look at them throughout the procedure.

The photos are important, as they reveal even minor differences between the two sides of the patient's face. I would not be able to operate without them. After studying the photos for the first of many times during the procedure, I read through the patient's original request form. This is the form they filled out in the original registration process, before we even met. Reading their words reminds me of the patient as a person, and the reason they visited me. It also allows me to re-check that what I'm planning to do is what they really wanted, and that the degree of change I'm aiming for is what they came in hoping for. At this point I often think of a cartoon I saw years ago that showed a customer in a restaurant ordering a porterhouse steak, giving the waiter precise instructions as to exactly how he wants it cooked. The waiter listens intently, bows and says, 'Of course,' then goes to the kitchen and barks the order to the chef, 'One porterhouse!' The plastic surgeon's set-up should be the reverse; the surgical plan may just say 'Face lift', but a wealth of detail lies behind those words.

By now the operating room door is closed, and any extraneous chatter about what we did on the weekend or what's going on in our lives ceases. We're like actors before a performance, locked away in our sealed world. We keep quiet while the anaesthetist completes their work so that we don't distract their attention, just as I expect not to be distracted during times of intense surgical focus.

I always appreciate the time after the patient has fallen asleep, under the spell of the anaesthetist's magic; the tube has been successfully placed and the patient's vital signs are settling. The anaesthetist then moves away from the patient to sit by the anaesthetic machine, and the time has come for the surgical team to move in. We no longer have to be aware of what the patient is feeling—hearing—so there's a healthy build up of tension as we quickly move into our routine.

Ergonomics are important to surgeons for operating well. Having comfortable access to the part of the face being worked on is essential. I use a foot-controlled, height-adjustable saddle stool designed for ergonomics and to minimise fatigue, and an operating table that has special narrow shoulders and a small headpiece, so I can sit close to the patient's head and avoid flexing my neck. The patient's position is adjusted by foot controls on the table, which I use almost subconsciously to maintain the ideal position of the operating field.

I tend to move the patient's position around quite a bit, so I can keep my back as straight as possible. The operating table I use is a modification of a dental chair, so it's designed to provide excellent access to the face and allow me to position the patient's head exactly as I want. Physically, the operation is a bit like running a marathon, so everything possible has to be done to avoid getting tired so you're still in good shape in the final hour.

The first thing I do to the patient is make surgical markings on their face with a fine surgical marking pen. Mostly, they're not necessary for the operation, but focusing intensely on them is another way of attuning my mind to the individual aspects of the procedure, as well as the individual nuances of the patient's face. Some markings, however, are critical. When I am planning for the removal of eyelid skin, this is measured to a fraction of a millimetre. Precision is so important that the eyelid markings are done with the patient still awake, opening and closing their eyes, for placement in the dynamic lid crease.

The next step, now that the patient is asleep, is to inject local anaesthetic solution into the part of the face I will be operating on first. This is done with surgical thought and precision, as the fluid facilitates the surgery. It is injected at the correct depth for the specific layers of the facial tissues where the dissection will be performed. Part of its role is to expand the tissues, which will make the dissection easier. Local anaesthetic is used even though the patient is asleep, as it reduces the body's response to the surgery by sparing the brain the sensation of pain. Another component of the injection fluid is adrenaline. This causes the blood vessels to constrict, which reduces the blood supply in the area I'll be operating on. You can see the skin blanching as the adrenaline starts to take effect.

The full response time for the adrenaline to be optimally effective is ten minutes, but that time passes quickly. The anaes-thetist, the anaesthetic nurse, the scrub nurse and the surgical assistant are all getting ready. I position the patient's head in the ideal way for operating, and the scrub nurse fixes back the patient's hair with hair product to keep it out of the way, applies antiseptic to the face and also to the abdomen—as a face lift usually includes some injection of fat into the face—then drapes the necessary areas before setting out the required instruments within easy reach. The surgical assistant then removes some fat from the patient's abdomen using a special cannula with many holes in it so the fine particles of fat collected can go into the centrifuge to separate the fat into its different components. After three minutes, the aspirated fat has split into its component layers; the true fat cells will be used, while the liquefied fat and fluid from the local anaesthetic will be discarded.

The first step in the procedure is usually to inject the lips with fat, to improve the volume and shape so they will match the fresher appearance of the patient's face. They need specific attention, as a face lift doesn't otherwise improve them. Through tiny incisions from a needle at each corner of the mouth, a fine cannula is used to thread in minute droplets of fat, gradually building up the volume. The amount of fat is monitored to ensure complete symmetry and that the volume is not excessive. Even a small excess here could ruin the natural look of the whole procedure before we have even started the face lift.

Now, at last, I can start the real operating. The next few hours will be a blend of routine operating interspersed with higher tension, critical moments, which occur when dissecting or placing sutures near to the nerve branches. They're actually my favourite moments.

Face lift surgery consists of three main stages. The first and most demanding of these is the dissection, or carefully cutting a path through the interior of the face to get to the area I want to operate on. This starts with an incision on the skin, which begins at the temple just above the ear and moves down past the front of the ear, under the earlobe and finishes up in the groove behind the ear. Precision is critical so that when it heals, it remains cleverly concealed in the subtle grooves immediately in the front of the ear. Usually it's possible to end the incision in the groove behind the ear, which is called the short scar technique, but if the patient has considerable laxity of the neck the incision will have to be extended further, from the top of the ear at the back and across the hairline. If this extended incision isn't done with absolute care, it may remain visible and the patient won't be able to shave his head or wear her hair up.

After the incision is made, I will be able to see into the interior of the face. From here on in, I'll be working three-dimensionally inside the patient's face. Imagine the patient lying there, with their face turned to the side away from you, the incision open down the front of their ear. Entering into that incision, I'll be moving under their skin, opening up various layers in the deeper anatomy of their face, as explained in earlier chapters, and travelling towards the centre of their face, which is where the correction will be. As we know, ageing occurs in the communication zone, close to the nose and mouth, which is a long distance from the incision at the ear. While it's a long and careful journey through the interior of the face, it is all familiar. As I dissect through, I will see the layers there, the spaces I'm looking for and the nerves I expect to see. I know the face intimately, and each landmark is both a comforting sight, and also a reminder that I've entered deeply personal territory, the face of the patient, so it's psychological and emotional territory as well. What I'm about to do, as I move forward, millimetre by millimetre, completing each step precisely, will affect their entire future life.

At the start of the journey—the incision—I separate the skin, with its layer of yellow subcutaneous fat attached to it, from the next layer, the SMAS, which has some white fibrous texture on its surface. Doing this involves surprisingly little bleeding, as the adrenaline injection and careful blood pressure control do their work. For some surgeons, this is as deep into the layers as they'll go. This was where early face lift surgeons like Suzanne Noël operated, and some still do, such as those who perform the skin stretching face lift.

But like most modern surgeons, I need to go deeper into the layers so I can use the patient's deeper anatomy to create a natural result. So, once I've separated the skin for about three centimetres forward of the incision, I move deeper into the face, through the underlying SMAS layer. Things change at this point—and not earlier—because the SMAS does not lift readily until this far forward, where it overlies the sub-SMAS spaces. For some surgeons, moving past this point is beyond their anatomical comfort zone and their skill, which is another reason they remain in what they consider 'safer' territory for themselves—essentially correcting the outer cheeks and attempting to tighten the skin of the inner cheeks and around the mouth by stretching it across from that point.

The dissection progresses, but I'm now underneath the SMAS and it, plus the skin above, form what is known as a composite flap. Essentially it's a complex and strong, blood-rich flap: Sushruta and Tagliacozzi would have loved to have seen this. Now I'm below the SMAS I also change the way I dissect: I begin to use blunt dissection, which means gently spreading blunt scissors and not cutting using a scalpel. This helps me find the spaces I'm looking for.

Once the spaces are clearly identified, I then enlarge them to their boundaries using a blunt dissection instrument and, for the largest space, the tip of my index finger is used with great sensitivity. These spaces are a wonder for a surgeon as there is absolutely no bleeding and minimal risk of injuring important structures when opening them properly. It reminds me of the games of Snakes and Ladders we played as children. Once the dissection lands in a space it is like landing on a ladder, as the reward allows you to move straight ahead to the front of the space, like getting to the top of the ladder. There are risks, just as in the game, but here it's not determined by chance. Instead, the surgeon controls the risk. Mainly, it's the presence of facial nerve branches, which lie closer to the ligaments of the face the further forward on the face you go. So I identify them, note their presence and keep away from them. To an inexperienced surgeon, the nerves and ligaments look similar but experience makes it easy to differentiate one from the other. Knowing where the nerves are in relation to the ligaments is tremendously empowering for the surgeon, just as familiarity with a track through the forest means a rally car driver can safely negotiate it at high speed, even if it is narrow and twisty and treacherous for the inexperienced.

The ligaments are like fibrous cords. These tiny white cords are my interest as they are really the reason I'm here. In a young patient the ligaments will look firm, but in an older patient they may already have weakened. Their role is to hold the SMAS in position, but I want to reposition the SMAS, so I have to release these ligaments first and then replace them with sutures (stitches) of my own, to hold the SMAS in the new position. This illustrates why it is so important for the surgeon to have a detailed understanding of facial anatomy.

The second stage of the face lift involves placing those sutures into the underside of the SMAS to reposition it close to the bone, as it was in youth (before the ligaments weakened). Surgically, this is the pay-off. Once the first suture is placed into the flap, I test the effect by drawing it tight. Immediately

I see the result on the skin above—a tremendous take-up of laxity on the side of the mouth, along with contouring over the cheek—across a much larger area of the face than you would expect from just a single suture. It shows the instant effect of these sutures. Every time I see this response it fills me with confidence. The dramatic and instantaneous removal of laxity, coming from deep within the face without any stretching on the overlying skin, is sensational.

The third stage in the face lift is about placing three or four more sutures in the right place to ensure an even correction. These sutures must endure so the patient can open her mouth, chew, bite and sleep on her face, so I use a strong permanent thread.

Even now, before the skin has been replaced into position, the benefit of the face lift in the central region of the face is obvious. I'm now ready to re-drape the skin over the newly re-contoured structure and trim any excess with precision, using very sharp scissors. To this day, I am constantly surprised by just how much excess skin there is to be removed.

Closure is simple with a forty-year-old because they still have good elasticity of their skin, but in an older patient with loose skin it takes some skill and patience to gather it all without little pleats being left. Finally, I close the incision in front of the ear and reset the earlobe into the correct position. It is critical that there not be even the slightest pull on the earlobe.

Now I can hand over to my assistant to complete the suturing of the incision. This allows me to take a break. There's no risk in that: a good assistant knows how to do everything necessary and you cannot detect any difference from his suturing to mine. Having a break during a long operation is critical to the maintenance of concentration. Just before handing over, however,

I gently turn the patient's head back to a central position in preparation for the injection of the local anaesthetic solution to the second side, so it has plenty of time to work while the closing is being performed of the first side. Now I can really see the improvement of the side I've just operated on by comparing it to the second side yet to be lifted. If I place my hand on the cheek and move it forwards, to mimic the effect of gravity, the unoperated side has extraordinary movement while the corrected side scarcely moves.

Finally, when the other side of the face has been operated on and surgery is complete, I review how the patient looks. On the way out of the theatre I gather the patient request form and the photographs from the wall bracket and have a second look to compare them with how the patient looks now. I wish the patients could see themselves at this stage before the onset of swelling. Instead, they'll have to wait several weeks as the swelling develops and then slowly subsides.

I leave the theatre tired but uplifted. It took so many years to develop the understanding, skills and experience to perform this quality face lift but all of that effort is justified when the patient looks really good. When I know that what I've done has met their hopes and more, I can't wait for the days to pass so they can see their new appearance. I glance back: fabulous.

A gift

I am now the person I should have been all along. It's a new opportunity to be who you really are. A gift. And it's so wonderful to just glide in like anyone else. Not being noticed is so much better than being noticed.

I've also noticed there's a feedback loop. I'm laughing more and people notice the difference, that I'm happy. I no longer wear a beanie because I no longer need comfort. I now want to help others.

This surgery is not smoke and mirrors for the rich and vain. It changes lives and gives self-worth. Our faces are the windows to who we are and often determine how we are received in the world. This is a vulnerability that is entirely unavoidable.

Sources

Alexander, C. (2007). *Faces of war*. Retrieved from
 www.smithsonianmag.com/history-archaeology/mask.html.
American Society for Aesthetic Plastic Surgery. (2011). *15th annual
 Cosmetic Surgery National Data Bank statistics*. Retrieved from
 www.surgery.org/sites/default/files/ASAPS-2011-Stats.pdf.
Beahrs, O H, Kiernan, P D & Hubert, J P Jnr. (1985). *An atlas of the surgical
 techniques of Oliver H. Beahrs*. Philadelphia, USA: WB Saunders.
Beauty does what money can't (2011, April 1). *The Age*. Retrieved from
 http://www.theage.com.au/lifestyle/beauty/beauty-does-what-money-
 cant-20110331-1cn9a.html.
Bloom, P. (2010) *How pleasure works: Why we like what we like*. London, UK:
 Vintage Books.
Carpue, J C. (1981). *An account of two successful operations for restoring a lost
 nose*. Birmingham, USA: Classics of Medicine Library. (Original work
 published 1816).
Castle, D J & Phillips, K A (Eds.). (2002). *Disorders of body image*. Petersfield,
 UK: Wrightson Biomedical Publishing.
Connell, B. (1978). Contouring the neck and rhytidoplasty by lipectomy and
 muscle sling. *Plastic and Reconstructive Surgery*, 61(3), 376-383.
Darwin, C. (1872). *The expression of the emotions in man and animals*. London,
 UK: John Murray.
De Quincey, T. (1821). *Confessions of an English opium eater*. London, UK:
 London Magazine.
Donahue, H. (2004). *Beautiful stranger: A memoir of obsession with perfection*.
 London, UK: Vision.
Duchenne de Boulogne, G. (1990). *The mechanism of human facial expression*
 (R A Cuthbertson, Ed. & Trans.). Cambridge, UK: Cambridge University
 Press & Editions de la Maison des sciences de l'homme.
Dwivedi, G & Dwivedi, S. (2007). Sushruta—the clinician—teacher par
 excellence. *The Indian Journal of Chest Diseases and Allied Sciences*, 49,
 243–244.

Eco, U. (2004). *On beauty: A history of a Western idea*. London, UK: Secker and Warburg.

Edmonds, A. (2010). *Pretty modern: Beauty, sex, and plastic surgery in Brazil*. Durham, USA: Duke University Press.

Ekman, P. (2001). *Telling lies*. New York, USA: WW Norton and Co. (Original work published 1985).

Ekman, P. (2003). *Emotions revealed: Understanding faces and feelings*. London, UK: Weidenfeld & Nicolson.

Elliott, A. (2008). *Making the cut: How cosmetic surgery is transforming our lives*. London, UK: Reaktion Books.

Ephron, N. (2006). *I feel bad about my neck*. New York, USA: Knopf Doubleday Publishing Group.

Etcoff, N L. (1994). Beauty and the beholder. *Nature, 368*, 186–187.

Ferrari, G. (1987). Public anatomy lessons and the carnival: The anatomy theatre of Bologna. *Past and Present, 117*(1), 50–106.

Frank, M G. (2001). Facial Expressions. In N Smelser & P Baltes (Eds.), *International encyclopedia of the social and behavioral sciences* (pp. 5230–5234). Oxford, UK: Pergamon.

Friel, M T, Shaw, R E, Trovato, M J & Owsley, J Q. (2010). The measure of face-lift patient satisfaction: the Owsley facelift satisfaction survey with a long-term follow-up study. *Plastic and Reconstructive Surgery, 126*(1), 245–257.

Furnas, D. (1989). The retaining ligaments of the cheek. *Plastic and Reconstructive Surgery, 83*(1), 11–16.

Gaston, V. (2010). *The naked face: Self-portraits*. Melbourne, Australia: National Gallery of Victoria.

Gerson, L. (2012). Plotinus. In E N Zalta (Ed.), *Stanford Encyclopedia of Philosophy*. Retrieved from http://plato.stanford.edu/archives/fall2012/entries/plotinus/.

Gibbs, D D. (1992). Sir Frederick Treves: Surgeon, author and medical historian. *Journal of the Royal Society of Medicine, 85*, 565–569.

Gillies, H D. (1920). *Plastic surgery of the face*. London, UK: Hodder and Stoughton.

Gillies, H D & Millard, D R Jr. (1957). *The principles and art of plastic surgery*. Boston, USA: Little, Brown.

Gladwell, M. (2002, August 5). The naked face. *The New Yorker*, pp. 38–49.

Gnudi, M T & Webster, J P. (1976). *The life and times of Gaspare Tagliacozzi, surgeon of Bologna, 1545–1599*. Los Angeles, USA: Zeitlin & Ver Brugge.

Goldwyn, R M. (1986). *Beyond appearance: Reflections of a plastic surgeon*. New York, USA: Dodd, Mead & Co.

González-Ulloa, M. (1980). The history of rhytidectomy. *Aesthetic Plastic Surgery, 4*(1), 1–45.

Greenwald, L. (2009). *Eye of the beholder: True stories of people with facial differences*. New York, USA: Kaplan Publishing.

Gregory, W K. (1929). *Our face from fish to man*. New York, USA: G.P. Putnam's Sons.

Gueguen, N, Jacob, C & Martin, A. (2009). Mimicry in social interaction: Its effect on human judgement and behaviour. *European Journal of Social Sciences*, *8*(12), 253–259.

Guerrero-Santos, J, Espaillat, L & Morales, F. (1974). Muscular lift in cervical rhytidoplasty. *Plastic and Reconstructive Surgery*, *54*(2), 127–131.

Hamermesh, D S. (2011). *Beauty pays: Why attractive people are more successful.* Princeton, USA: Princeton University Press.

Hamra, S T. (1993). *Composite rhytidectomy.* St Louis, USA: Quality Medical Publishing.

Hobday, V. (2006). *A body of evidence: An art historical perspective on eighteenth and nineteenth century wax anatomical models.* [Master's thesis]. Melbourne, Australia: University of Melbourne School of Art History.

Hogarth, W. (1955). *The analysis of beauty.* Oxford, UK: Clarendon Press. (Original work published 1753).

Huxley, A. (1952). *Brave new world.* London, UK: Vanguard.

International Society of Aesthetic Plastic Surgery. (2011). *ISAPS international survey of aesthetic/cosmetic procedures performed in 2010.* Retrieved from www.isaps.org/files/html-contents/ISAPS-Procedures-Study-Results-2011.pdf.

Joseph, J. (1987). *Rhinoplasty and facial plastic surgery with a supplement on mammaplasty and other operations in the field of plastic surgery of the body: An atlas and textbook* (S Milstein, Trans.). Phoenix, USA: Columella Press. (Original work published 1931).

Kahneman, D. (2012). *Thinking fast and slow.* Melbourne, Australia: Penguin Books.

Kosowski, T R, McCarthy, C, Reavey, P L, Scott, A M, Wilkins, E G, Cano, S J, Klassen, A F, Carr, N, Cordeiro, P G & Pusic, A L. (2009). A systematic review of patient-reported outcome measures after facial cosmetic surgery and/or nonsurgical facial rejuvenation. *Plastic and Reconstructive Surgery*, *123*(6), 1819–1827.

Lavater, J K. (1853). *Essays on physiognomy: Designed to promote the knowledge and love of mankind* (T Holcroft, Trans.). London, UK: William Tegg & Co. (Original work published 1775–78).

Lemmon, M L & Hamra, S T. (1980). Skoog rhytidectomy: A 5-year experience with 577 patients. *Plastic and Reconstructive Surgery*, *65*(3), 283–297.

Little, A & Perrett, D. (2002). Putting beauty back in the eye of the beholder. *The Psychologist*, *15*(1), 28–32.

Little, J W. (2000a). Volumetric perceptions in midfacial aging with altered priorities for rejuvenation. *Plastic and Reconstructive Surgery*, *105*(1), 252–266.

Little, J W. (2000b). Three dimensional rejuvenation of the midface: Volumetric resculpture by malar imbrication. *Plastic and Reconstructive Surgery*, *105*(1), 267–285.

Liu, T S & Owsley, J Q. (2012). Long-term results of face lift surgery: Patient photographs compared with patient satisfaction ratings. *Plastic and Reconstructive Surgery*, *129*(1), 253–62.

Livio, M. (2002). *The golden ratio.* New York, USA: Broadway Books.

Macdonald, A. (1993). Rogers v Whitaker: Duty of disclosure. *Bioethics Research Notes, 5*(3).

MacDonald, H. (2005). *Human remains: Episodes in human dissection.* Melbourne, Australia: Melbourne University Publishing.

McDowell, F. (1969). Ancient ear-lobe and rhinoplastic operations in India. *Plastic and Reconstructive Surgery, 43*(5), 515–618.

McDowell, F. (1969). Development of plastic surgery from ancient times to the end of the eighteenth century. *Plastic and Reconstructive Surgery, 43*(6), 618.

McDowell, F. (1976). History of rhinoplasty. *Aesthetic Plastic Surgery, 1*(1), 321–48.

Macgregor, F C. (1990). Facial disfigurement: Problems and management of social interaction and implications for mental health. *Aesthetic Plastic Surgery, 14*(1), 249–257.

McLeave, H. (1961). *McIndoe: Plastic surgeon.* London, UK: Frederick Muller.

McNeill, D. (1998). *The face: A natural history.* Boston, USA: Little, Brown.

Maltz, M. (1936). *New faces, new futures: Rebuilding character with plastic surgery.* New York, USA: Richard R Smith.

Maltz, M. (1954). *Doctor Pygmalion.* London, UK: Museum Press Limited.

Mazzola, R. (2009). Suzanne Noël: Pioneer in aesthetic surgery and founder of the Soroptimist Europe. *ISAPS Newsletter, March–June,* 18–19.

Mendelson, B C. (2007, October 21). ASAPS Oration. *Thirty-first annual conference of the Australasian Society of Aesthetic Plastic Surgery.* Adelaide, Australia.

Mendelson, B C. (2008). Advances in understanding the surgical anatomy of the face. In M Eisennmann-Klein & C Neuhann-Lorenz (Eds.), *Innovations in Plastic and Aesthetic Surgery* (pp. 145–149). Heidelberg, Germany: Springer Verlag.

Mendelson, B C. (2009). *Understanding facelift anatomy.* [DVD recording].

Mendelson, B C, Muzaffar, A R & Adams, W P Jr. (2002). Surgical anatomy of the midcheek and malar mounds. *Plastic and Reconstructive Surgery, 110*(3), 885–896.

Mendelson, B C & Wong, C H. (2012). Changes of the facial skeleton with ageing: Implications and clinical applications in facial rejuvenation. *Aesthetic Plastic Surgery, 36*(4), 753–760

Moebius Syndrome Foundation. (2007). *Home page.* Retrieved from www. moebiussyndrome.com.

Morselli, P G. (1993). The minotaur syndrome: Plastic surgery of the facial skeleton. *Aesthetic Plastic Surgery, 17*(2), 99–102.

Morselli, P G. (2008). Maxwell Maltz, psychocybernetic plastic surgeon, and personal reflections on dysmorphopathology. *Aesthetic Plastic Surgery, 32*(3), 485–495.

Noël, S. (2011). *Aesthetic surgery and its social significance* (R McClure, Trans.). Unpublished translation. (Original work published 1929).

Orwell, G. (1949). *Nineteen eighty-four.* London, UK: Secker and Warburg.

Owsley, J Q Jr. (1983). SMAS–platysma face lift. *Plastic and Reconstructive Surgery, 71*(4), 573–576.

Patil, B. (2003). *The meaning of depression and malaise seen from the perspective of Hinduism*. Retrieved from www.healthpastoral.org/events/18conference/patil.htm.

Perfect face dimensions measured. (2009, December 18). *BBC News Online*. Retrieved from http://news.bbc.co.uk/2/hi/8421076.stm.

Perrett, D I, May, K A & Yoshikawa, S. (1994). Facial shape and judgements of female attractiveness. *Nature, 368*, 239–242.

Pound, R. (1964). *Gillies: Surgeon extraordinary*. London, UK: Michael Joseph.

Powell, N. & Humphreys, B. (1984). *Proportions of the aesthetic face*. New York, USA: Thieme Stratton Inc.

Powers, R. (2006). *The echo maker*. London, UK: William Heinemann.

Queen Mary's Hospital. (2012). *The Gillies archives*. Sidcup, UK: Queen Mary's Hospital. Retrieved from www.gilliesarchives.org.uk.

Quill, E. (2009). It's written all over your face. *Science News, 175*(2), 24–28.

Rank, B K. (1958). Fact and fiction of facial plastic surgery. *Medical Journal of Australia*.

Regnault, P & Stephenson, K L. (1971). Dr Suzanne Noël: The first woman to do esthetic surgery. *Plastic and Reconstructive Surgery, 48*(2), 133–139.

Rhode, D L. (2010). *The beauty bias: The injustice of appearance in life and law*. New York, USA: Oxford University Press USA.

Rhodes, G, Hickford, C & Jeffery, L. (2000). Sex-typicality and attractiveness: Are supermale and superfemale faces super-attractive? *British Journal of Psychology, 91*(1), 125–140.

Rogers, B O. (1976–78). The development of aesthetic plastic surgery: a history. *Aesthetic Plastic Surgery, 1*(1), 3–24.

Rogers, B O. (1986). John Orlando Roe—not Jacques Joseph—the father of aesthetic rhinoplasty. *Aesthetic Plastic Surgery, 10*(2), 63–88.

Sacks, O. (2012). *The mind's eye*. London, UK: Picador.

Skoog, T. (1974). *Plastic surgery: new methods and refinements*. Philadelphia, USA: WB Saunders.

Society for Neuroscience. (2012, October 14). New research reveals more about how the brain processes facial expression and emotions. [Press release]. Retrieved from www.sfn.org/index.aspx?pagename=news_101412_faces.

Stephenson, K. (1976–78). The history of blepharoplasty to correct blepharochalasis. *Aesthetic Plastic Surgery, 1*(1), 177–194.

Stofman, G M, Neavin, T S, Ramineni, P M & Alford, A. Better sex from the knife? An intimate look at the effects of cosmetic surgery on sexual practices. *Aesthetic Surgery Journal, 26*(1), 12–17.

Swan, N (Presenter) & Rossell, S (Guest). (2010, September 20). Body dysmorphic disorder. [Radio broadcast]. In B. Seega (Producer), *The health report*. Sydney, Australia: ABC Radio National.

Swanson, E. (2011). Outcome analysis in 93 facial rejuvenation patients treated with a deep-plane face lift. *Plastic and Reconstructive Surgery, 127*(2), 823–834.

Taschen, A (Ed.). (2005). *Aesthetic surgery*. Cologne, Germany: Taschen.

Thornhill, R & Gangestad, S W. (1999). Facial attractiveness. *Trends in Cognitive Sciences*, 3(12), 452–460.

Trumble, A. (2004). *A brief history of the smile*. Sydney, Australia: Allen & Unwin.

UCLA Health System. (2012). *UCLA Operation Mend*. Retrieved from http://operationmend.ucla.edu

United Nations Department of Economic and Social Affairs. (2001). *World Population Ageing: 1950–2050*. New York, USA: United Nations.

Valenzano, D R, Mennucci, A, Tartarelli, G & Cellerino, A. (2006). Shape analysis of female facial attractiveness. *Vision Research*, 46(8–9), 1282–1291.

Willi, C H. (1926). *Facial rejuvenation*. London, UK: Cecil Palmer.

Willi, C H. (1949). *The face and its improvement by aesthetic plastic surgery*. London, UK: Melville Press Limited.

Winston, J S, O'Doherty, J, Kilner, J M, Perrett, D I & Dolan, R J. (2007). Brain systems for assessing facial attractiveness. *Neuropsychologia*, 45(1), 195–206.

Wolf, N. (1991). *The beauty myth*. New York, USA: William Morrow and Company.

Young, M. (2011, July 29). The ugliness penalty. *New York*. Retrieved from http://nymag.com/news/intelligencer/the-ugliness-penalty-2011-8/.

Acknowledgements

I want to express my heartfelt thanks to the many patients who unhesitatingly offered their personal stories. Their openness was the stimulus for this book and their experiences, expressed in their words, are the message. I apologise to the patients whose stories were not included by the editor, only to minimise repetition. Hopefully, they will be consoled by another patient's story that is similar—after all, most people do have a similar experience.

Of course no man is an island and every surgeon has a debt to his teachers, as I have in particular to the Mayo Clinic surgeons: Ollie Beahrs for his feeling for surgical anatomy and magician's mastery with the tissues, and Don McIlrath for pushing us uncompromisingly to be real surgeons. In plastic surgery at the Mayo Clinic, John Woods, for his humanity, James Masson for his elegance, PG Arnold for his boldness, and in New York, Sherrell Aston for his energy and loyal support. Later on it was Bruce Connell and Robert Flowers for bringing the surgery up to their high aesthetic standards.

I apologise to the patients, hopefully few, especially those in my earlier years, who tolerated results that were not of today's standard, as well as those with a high aesthetic eye who drew my attention to aspects of appearance that I had not yet appreciated. But thanks always to the patients for expressing their gratitude and opening my awareness to the potential, and therefore my responsibility each time I operate, to enrich each patient's quality of life. This was made possible through the special care and support given by the select few anaesthetists who have worked with me, my dedicated office staff over the years and especially Terry Tiong, my longstanding surgical assistant, who I suspect could operate when my back is turned!